Concierge Medicine

Concierge Medicine

A New System to Get the Best Healthcare

STEVEN D. KNOPE, M.D.

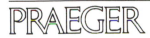 PRAEGER

Westport, Connecticut
London

Library of Congress Cataloging-in-Publication Data

Knope, Steven D.
   Concierge medicine : a new system to get the best healthcare / Steven D. Knope.
     p. ; cm.
   Includes bibliographical references and index.
   ISBN: 978–0–313–35477–9 (alk. paper)
   1. Medicine—Practice. 2. Medical care. 3. Health care rationing.
   [DNLM: 1. Comprehensive Health Care. 2. Physician's Practice
Patterns—economics. 3. Insurance, Health, Reimbursement—economics.
4. Privatization—organization & administration. W 87 K72c 2008] I. Title.
   R728.K57 2008
   610.68—dc22   2008002507

British Library Cataloguing in Publication Data is available.

Library of Congress Catalog Card Number: 2008002507
ISBN: 978–0–313–35477–9

First published in 2008

Praeger Publishers, 88 Post Road West, Westport, CT 06881
An imprint of Greenwood Publishing Group, Inc.
www.praeger.com

Printed in the United States of America

The paper used in this book complies with the
Permanent Paper Standard issued by the National
Information Standards Organization (Z39.48–1984).

10 9 8 7 6 5 4 3 2

Contents

Introduction

I am a board-certified internist and graduate of the Cornell Medical College. I am also what is called a concierge physician. I take care of people who desire excellence in traditional medicine and who want guidance regarding the protection of their most precious asset—their health.

By paying me, my patients are making an investment in their health. They want a return on that investment. They want their health to be protected. They want to feel better. Many want to look better. They want improvements in their sexual function. They want greater productiveness, alertness, and stamina. They want to live as long as possible. They want quality and value added to their years. They want to get the most out of their lives.

As a concierge physician, I am available to my patients by beeper or telephone, 24 hours per day, 7 days per week. I care for my patients when they are hospitalized. I do not turn their care over to a "hospitalist" when they become seriously ill. That is the time when a patient needs his doctor the most. You don't want an unknown doctor taking care of you when you are critically ill. When you choose a doctor, what you are selecting is his mind, his training, and his experience.

Similarly, when you read the latest article on improving your health, you often need a filter for medical information. There is some good health information on the Internet and in health magazines, but there is a lot of junk out there as well. When you just want an answer to your health questions, wouldn't it be nice to be able to call a doctor and be seen promptly to discuss your concerns?

When my patients call for an appointment, they are seen on the same day. There are no long waits in the waiting room or the examination room. When necessary, I have found world-class specialists for my patients. I've boarded private jets to fly with them for their consultations. I make house calls. I meet my patients in the emergency room (ER) when they have an emergency. In short, I am a modern-day Marcus Welby, M.D., with all the benefits of the latest advances in medical technology.

How can this be? How can my patients get this kind of care? In a recent poll by WebMD, one-third of Americans said the U.S. healthcare system was broken and should be completely rebuilt. However, my patients and many others in concierge practices all over the country have found a way around the broken system. They have invested in their own healthcare by paying the doctor directly for his services. The result is a huge return on their investment.

If you think concierge medicine is only for the wealthy, read on. There are concierge plans now available for virtually all middle-income people in America. Concierge medicine is not one form of practice but a spectrum of individualized medical services offered at varying prices. In this book, I will show you why concierge medicine is worth exploring and how you can work concierge medicine care into your budget.

THE BENEFITS OF TIME AND ACCESS

Like an old-fashioned doctor, I run my own private practice. I do not work for an HMO. I do not take managed care contracts. I do not accept government dollars in the form of Medicare. However, as you will read, I used to practice this kind of medicine. As the Chief of Medicine at a large community hospital, I saw thirty to forty patients every day. I saw the poor care that patients receive in high volume practices. I presided over review boards that examined medical mistakes. I worked fervently to reform the system. I fought the good fight. However, in spite of my idealism and efforts, I failed to change the system for the better.

What I ultimately learned was that systems change in our culture when market forces drive change. Despite my previous naiveté, the same holds true in medicine. Consumers force changes by demanding better services. It was my patients who ultimately convinced me to open a concierge practice. This allowed me the freedom to act as their advocate and do what I do best: practice medicine.

I have structured my practice so that I now have more time with each patient. Time, as you will read later, is absolutely essential for good medical care. I no longer see thirty patients per day. I now see only twelve to fifteen. There is no substitute for time in solving complex medical problems. As medicine becomes more and more complicated, *more time*, not less, is needed to find the best solution for a patient.

As patients become more sophisticated and have greater access to medical information on the Internet, they have more questions. They need more of a doctor's time to understand their medical issues. A healthcare delivery system that operates like a fast-food chain, dispensing quick fixes as if they were Happy Meals, does nothing to provide excellence in medicine. It doesn't take care of people. Our current superficial and fragmented approach to medical care is driven not by the pursuit of quality; it is driven by financial pressures from third-party payers and a Medicare system in trouble.

In a concierge arrangement, the third-party payment to the doctor is either minimized or eliminated. This places the financial responsibility on the patient. The patient becomes a consumer. They can shop for the doctor who offers the best care at the right price. It puts the doctor back in the role of patient advocate. It fosters one of the most therapeutic and useful tools in healing, something called the doctor–patient relationship. And it allows the investor to evaluate his return on investment.

A PERSONAL INVESTMENT

To accept the notion that good medical care requires a personal investment of money and time requires a paradigm shift. For people who run businesses or have wealth, this is not much of an adjustment. Businessmen and women pay expert advisors and professionals to protect their assets every day of their lives. They understand the value of having a good attorney and a good accountant. The cost of these professionals is simply the cost of doing business. Good professionals keep them out of trouble. Expert professional help is not considered a waste of money.

For those who do not own and operate businesses but work for others for a living, the concept of investing in professional consultants may take a little getting used to. In this book I will show you in very practical terms how you can afford to invest in your health and still stay within your budget.

The most important thing to understand is that the real paradigm shift comes not in accepting the idea that good medicine costs money but that *your health is an asset that deserves your investment*. I am going to tell you how to protect and grow your health using the expertise of a concierge doctor. Since you don't, or at least shouldn't, neglect your financial assets, I am going to suggest that you treat your health with similar care.

In this book, I am going to show you that the value of your health portfolio can be easily measured. I will then tell you how you can invest wisely to make your health grow so that you can get more out of life. I hope that after reading these pages you will be convinced that your health should be treated with *at least* as much care as your financial investments.

WHAT I'VE LEARNED FROM RICH GUYS WITH HEART DISEASE

Though people often say, "If you have your health, you have everything," most do not behave as if this were true. Most people take better care of their "stuff" than they do of their bodies. They do not have expert medical backup in the event of a crisis. They do not have a personal relationship with their doctor. They lack good information on wellness, and they don't know how to achieve it.

Several years ago, I was asked by a local specialty hospital to speak to a group of twenty prominent businessmen who had all suffered either a heart attack or had a bypass operation. These catastrophic events had shaken these financial achievers to their core. They met every Thursday over lunch to attend a support group at the hospital. They invited various medical experts to address topics on how they might stay healthy, prevent recurrent heart disease, and deal with the limitations created by their serious illnesses.

As I prepared for this talk, I decided to get a bit bold with the title. I wanted to get their attention. The first slide on my PowerPoint presentation read, "What I've Learned from Rich Guys with Heart Disease." There was an uncomfortable laughter as I put the first slide up. However, they knew immediately what I was talking about. Much of the predicament that they found themselves in was due to a *lack of investment* in their health.

What I've learned from fifteen years of clinical practice is that people of all socioeconomic levels take better care of their money than they do of their health! They invest more time and money protecting their financial assets than they do in their most precious of assets. Many of my patients would never do anything as irresponsible as failing to change their car's oil every 5,000 miles, yet they think nothing of pouring "junk" into their own gas tanks. They schedule regular maintenance of their home's roof, but they do not exercise. Somehow, it's just not worth the investment.

The results of poor investment strategies in the financial arena can be devastating. If you fail to mind your business, you can end up in bankruptcy court. However, there is a more ominous form of poverty that can affect *any person*, regardless of socioeconomic status. If you only concentrate on making money and fail to invest in your health, you can end up a rich person in a dilapidated body. Disease and illness create a kind of destitution even more devastating than bankruptcy. In terms of quality of life, health is the great equalizer.

IF IT'S GOOD ENOUGH FOR MY EMPLOYEES, IT'S GOOD ENOUGH FOR ME!

Early on in my career, when I was still accepting HMO insurance plans, a wealthy entrepreneur came to see me to establish care. This man had built a mom-and-pop business into a $17 million enterprise over just two decades. When I looked at his chart, I saw that he was insured by a local HMO known for its cut-rate services.

I was amazed that this intelligent man would invest so little in his own healthcare. I asked why he didn't get private insurance for himself and his family. He replied, "If the plan is good enough for my employees, it's good enough for me." His heart was in the right place, but the HMO this entrepreneur had enrolled in was good enough for neither himself nor his employees.

I looked further into his medical history. He had belonged to an out-of-state HMO prior to moving to Tucson. While under the care of this HMO, he went in for a routine surgery. There was a major complication during the operation. He nearly bled to death. He had suffered anoxic brain damage during the surgery. When I ordered complex neuropsychological testing on this gentleman, serious cognitive deficits became apparent. It was only a matter of time before this disaster would catch up to him.

As it turned out, he had gotten exactly what he paid for. He drove the finest of automobiles and lived in a beautiful home. However, he got his healthcare at a fast-food restaurant. If you have any concern for your health as an asset, you don't buy raw sushi from a street vendor, and you don't get your medical care from a cut-rate HMO. This man was a brilliant entrepreneur, but he was penny wise and pound foolish with his most precious asset.

EXECUTIVE PHYSICALS

Not all people are so careless with their health. Some people even travel to places like the Mayo Clinic once a year for an "executive physical." During these comprehensive evaluations, they have their body parts parceled out and examined by multiple specialists. They have a colonoscopy done by a gastroenterologist, a stress test done by a cardiologist, and a blood test examined by an internist. At the end of this process, they get a clean bill of health written on a fancy piece of letterhead. When they return to their hometown, they at least know that they are free of immediate health threats.

There is nothing wrong with an executive physical at a world-class clinic, if you can afford it. The problem is that when you get back home, you do not have the same level of care. You don't have the Mayo Clinic in your own backyard should you develop a problem. Equally important, by getting your healthcare elsewhere, you have not built a relationship with a trusted medical advisor. You do not have a personal physician. This is why many of my concierge patients have switched their care from the Mayo Clinic or the Scripps Clinic to a concierge arrangement. They want continuity. They want my time and availability. They want someone whom they can call at 2 o'clock in the morning with chest pain. If they need a subspecialist at the Mayo Clinic, they can always get a consultation there. However, if you can't afford to fly to the Mayo Clinic but have a good concierge physician, he can find an excellent specialist in your area. As your personal doctor, he is a healthcare advocate.

Even after spending thousands of dollars at exclusive executive clinics to screen for disease, people will often leave with little or no under-standing of what health or wellness is all about. They may be free of disease, but this does not necessarily mean that they are healthy. Wellness is more than the mere absence of disease. Wellness is an optimal state of functioning. Many people do not understand that wellness is something that only you can create for yourself. Creating wellness takes time, knowledge, and professional guidance.

WEALTH EQUALS FREEDOM

Good health should be viewed as a form of capital, like financial wealth. What is the real value of financial wealth? Why do people without wealth play the lottery? What's the big deal about money? Malcolm Forbes said, "He with the most toys in the end wins." I disagree. Toys are fun. But the real reason to have wealth is that it *buys freedom*. It buys choices. When you are financially stronger, you have more options in life. Your time does not belong to someone else. You are not chained to a job that you hate. You can travel. Money can be used to do many wonderful things, not only for yourself and your family, but also for the world around you.

In my world, health is the most important capital of all. I say this because I know how people suffer when they are in poor health. I've taken care of people worth hundreds of millions of dollars who have been in very poor health; I've cared for middle-class men and women in robust health. Given the choice, I'd take the latter. With great health, you have freedom from disease and disability. You have the freedom of living an active lifestyle, even late into your life.

When your health is poor, your life is dominated by doctor visits, hospital admissions, surgeries and endless tests. Your time is literally taken away from you in an effort to prolong your life. You are burdened with pain, discomfort, worry, and the inability to enjoy the simple pleasures of life. *When you become sick, you become a passive object in a system that does things to you.* If there is any way to avoid this fate, it makes sense to do so, especially when such a small investment is all that is needed.

TAKING RESPONSIBILITY FOR YOUR HEALTH

It will be no surprise to you when I acknowledge that our current healthcare system is in disarray. Good healthcare is no longer a given. Due to the erosion of the medical system from many outside forces, you can no longer assume that once you enter the system you will be well cared for. You cannot simply pay an insurance premium anymore and expect good healthcare. You must take things into your own hands. If you want good care, you are going to have to pay for it yourself.

Sadly, the once-great spirit of the medical profession that drove the unparalleled quality of our medical care in the United States has been broken. The profession has lost its heart. Third-party payers and government bureaucracies now run the financial and professional lives of most doctors. Many doctors have become little more than disgruntled employees of HMOs, insurance companies, or the federal government.

Most of the doctors whom I know are unhappy. They look at me in amazement when I say that I still love the practice of medicine. They would leave the profession in a heartbeat if they could. Several of my colleagues in Tucson recently sold an equity interest in a local managed care clinic that bought their practice. They were each given a buyout of $3 million. They were so disheartened by the system that this was all it took for dozens of doctors, in the prime of their professional lives, to opt out of a lifetime of professional investment in medicine. I wouldn't quit medicine if I got $3 million tomorrow. I like medicine.

To maintain their income with falling reimbursement, most doctors simply run faster and faster. They see more and more patients every day, spending less and less time with each one of them. They behave as if they are mice on a running wheel. I don't know about you, but when I get sick, I am going to want to be cared for by someone who is strong, smart, and well rested. I want a doctor who is still in love with the practice of medicine, not a mouse in a cage. It's an inconvenience if my mechanic hates his life and his job; I can always buy a new car if he screws up. However, I want my doctor to love his work. I want him to have the time and energy to care.

YOUR HEALTH PORTFOLIO

The rest of this book will be devoted to sharing with you what I know about investing in your health. After reading this book, you will have more options. It is my hope that you will look at healthcare in an entirely different way. You will view your health as an asset. It is my hope that this will also change the way that you view the health of your family and loved ones. Concierge medicine isn't just for rich guys. The principles of finding a competent physician, exercising, and eating well apply to men, women, and children of all ages and backgrounds.

I will explain the phenomenon of concierge medicine, which is gaining new adherents every day. The success of concierge medicine lies in the fact that it restores choices—choices for the patient and choices for the doctor.

I will teach you how to find a doctor who can meet your needs despite our broken healthcare system.

You will understand that there are three critical components of comprehensive healthcare: medical care, exercise, and nutrition. Each of these components should be in place if you wish to get the most out of your life. After reading these pages, you will understand what wellness is and what it is not. You will learn that the value of your health portfolio can be measured objectively just like your financial portfolio. You can assign a net worth to your present health. I will show you how you can make sound investments to grow your health over time.

I will devote an entire chapter to a critically important investment tool called exercise, even if the subject makes you cringe at the moment. I will tell you how to create greater strength and endurance. I will explain how to do it efficiently. I will show you how a small investment of time will generate large returns on your investment. I will demystify the subject of diets and nutrition and help you understand how to optimally fuel your body.

WHY I PRACTICE CONCIERGE MEDICINE

When I was in medical school, I kept reminding myself that the sacrifices I was making would some day translate into people leading greater lives. Ultimately, I don't care what people do with their time. This is their choice. However, the idea that I could help patch people up, help make them healthier, and get them back to doing what makes them unique human beings has always been fun for me.

I get as much satisfaction out of helping my patients as they get out of me. It is a great profession! I love practicing concierge medicine. I like helping motivated people invest in their most precious asset. I enjoy watching someone's health portfolio grow. I enjoy caring most for people who want to thrive, as opposed to those who want merely to survive. After honing my skills over the past decade and a half, I hope that the information I will share with you in these pages will make you healthier. I hope that your improvement in health will spread to your friends and your family. It is my hope that after reading this book, you will have the tools to create a better and richer life.

CHAPTER 1

Who Killed Marcus Welby, M.D.?

For a generation, Dr. Marcus Welby was the Hollywood embodiment of the caring personal physician. The series *Marcus Welby, M.D.* was a huge commercial success and lasted seven years on primetime television. During the entire year of 1970, it was the number-one TV show in the nation, viewed every week by one in four American families.

Doctor dramas have always captured the imagination of television viewers, starting with *Dr. Kildare* in the 1960s, *M*A*S*H** in the 1970s and 1980s and *Grey's Anatomy* in the 2000s. However, what was unique to *Marcus Welby, M.D.* was the show's focus on the doctor–patient relationship. It was not just how Welby managed the disease that was important; it was how he *treated* his patients.

Welby was in solo practice. He was not an employee of a large group practice. He did not work for an HMO (Health Maintenance Organization). The success of his practice was based on the kind of doctor he was and the quality of the medicine that he practiced. From a business perspective, medical practices in Welby's day were built on referrals from existing patients as well as from other physicians who respected the doctor. Things are different for most doctors today. Most patients now pick a doctor from an insurance list.

The show was quite innovative at the time in that it addressed the fact that about 30 percent of all visits to the doctor concern problems that do not fit the biomedical model. In other words, the complaint of the patient does not result in a pathological diagnosis for which medicine is dispensed or surgery is recommended. Patients often seek the help of their doctors for psychological, behavioral, or social problems that may manifest in physical symptoms. *Marcus Welby, M.D.* spotlighted problems such as depression, substance abuse, and even sexual assault.

By being kind to his patients, Welby was not just being a nice guy. He was actually being a more effective physician. He built trust and gained the confidence of his patients. As a result, they were more likely to confide in him, as well as to comply with his treatment recommendations. Additionally, when patients did have life-threatening medical illnesses, his compassion became an important part of the healing process.

Like all television series, *Marcus Welby, M.D.* came to an end, finally taken off the air in 1976. Interestingly, at about the same time, the real Marcus Welbys of the world were also beginning to vanish from the medical landscape. As private practice became increasingly more difficult to manage, many doctors began joining large group practices or multispecialty groups. Fewer young doctors seemed willing to hang out their own shingles after finishing their training. The face of medicine was changing rapidly, and not necessarily for the better.

What happened to the real Dr. Welbys of America? Were these independent practitioners euthanized by a modern culture that no longer valued the personal physician? Did generalists become obsolete with the emergence of subspecialty medicine? Perhaps these private doctors met a more sinister fate. Just who killed Marcus Welby, M.D.?

THE CRIMINAL INVESTIGATION

If law enforcement officers had been summoned to investigate the disappearance of Dr. Welby on primetime television, they would have started by gathering information about any enemies Welby might have had. They would have interviewed his friends and family members for clues and talked with his young associate, Dr. Steven Kiley, to find out if anyone had a motive to snuff the good doctor.

If you asked any practicing physician what happened to the real Dr. Welbys of our time, you would get a quick and simple answer. Solo practitioners were faced with three threats to their financial and professional survival beginning in the 1970s: the hostile takeover of the medical profession by a burgeoning HMO industry, a national malpractice crisis, and a failing Medicare system that cut physician reimbursement so low that doctors could no longer afford to spend time with their patients.

Each of these developments was a major blow to private doctors. What was more, all of these threats were occurring simultaneously. Suddenly, all the rules of the game were changing. What had been a cottage industry of small, private medical practices was soon being transformed by the "businessification" of medicine. Doctors, who previously had no need for sophisticated business skills, were suddenly negotiating contracts with MBAs for their very financial survival. In this process, doctors were easy marks. They did not even speak the language of business. Their arrogance prevented them from seeing what they did not understand.

Major insurance companies began controlling large patient "panels," thus controlling the money that flowed to physicians. After taking control of the purse strings, these corporations then negotiated with the doctor regarding how much he was to be paid, how much time he could afford to spend with his patients, and what tests he could or could not order without corporate approval. The doctor was becoming an unwitting employee of third-party payers. In addition, patients could see the doctor only if he was on their insurance plan. As for the U.S. government's role in his undoing, the Medicare bureaucrats could set and later reduce the doctor's rates, and there wasn't a thing he could do about it.

To the CEOs of corporate medicine on Wall Street, doctors were interchangeable cogs in a business machine, just like the employees at a burger franchise. One doctor was no different from another. Differences in the education, skill, or training of a physician were minimized or discounted altogether by the suits. An internist was an internist, a pediatrician was a pediatrician. If the doctors didn't like the terms of the contract, they could go elsewhere. The language used to address medical doctors was even changed by the business administrators to diminish the social stature and professional power of the doctor. In the new business model, physicians were no longer even referred to as "doctors." Instead, HMOs and business executives started referring to doctors as "providers." I wonder if the famous TV show would have had many viewers had it been called *Marcus Welby, Provider*.

The impact of these changes on patients was profound. Without understanding why, they began to notice that the doctor was less available to them. He seemed more hurried. He had less time to listen to them and deal with them as people. Whereas previously they could have gotten an appointment to see their doctor on relatively short notice, they now had to wait weeks—as if they had been overbooked on some budget airline. It became almost impossible to talk to the doctor by phone to get an answer to a quick question. The difference between the TV portrayal of Marcus Welby's brand of medicine and that of the real world became rather striking. According to the Museum of Broadcast Communications, Robert Young (the actor who played Welby) was once attending a conference of family practice doctors. One of them said, "You're getting us all into hot water. Our patients tell us we're not as nice to them as Doctor Welby is to his patients." Young replied, "Maybe you're not."

In 1994, a year after beginning work for a group of five internists in Tucson, I decided to leave the safety of the group and open my own private practice. I did not like the pressures exerted on me by my employers to accept the new world order. I did not like being a cog in a wheel.

Many of my colleagues at the hospital warned me about my decision to go it alone. They said I was "too idealistic." They said that by striking out on my own I would be losing the protection of the pack when it came to contract negotiations. They projected that I would soon be eaten by the corporate predators. All around me, doctors were forming larger and larger groups in an attempt to maintain some level of control at the bargaining table. They hired MBAs to manage their practices. However, becoming a member of a large group just didn't fit my personality. I was too independent. I didn't like herding patients in and out of my office like cattle. In my view, it wasn't good medicine and it wasn't fair to my patients. It was certainly not rewarding for me.

In retrospect, starting my own practice was the most important professional decision I've ever made. It was the first of several decisions that would allow me to blaze my own trail in medicine and create a practice which would be more akin to Welby's. My patients noticed the difference immediately. My smaller and more intimate office made them feel more at home. They truly appreciated the differences that came from more personalized care. As you will read later, this decision came with a price, but it was worth it.

THREATENED WITH EXTINCTION

If we look at what has happened to the practice of medicine in just one generation, there is convincing evidence that internists and family practice doctors in America are indeed a dying breed. Primary care doctors have been officially placed on the medical endangered species list. In fact, it is not just that solo internists and family practitioners are vanishing. Very few doctors want to practice primary care medicine at all anymore. Being a primary care doc-in-the-box at a large clinic is just not very appealing. Fewer medical school graduates are opting for careers in internal medicine or family practice.

If this trend continues, the loss of primary care medicine could have serious implications for the delivery of healthcare to our aging population over the next few decades. The American College of Physicians recently issued a position paper stating, "Primary care, the backbone of the nation's health care system, is at grave risk of collapse." On August 31, 2006, shortly after this proclamation, the *New England Journal of Medicine* published an article entitled "Primary Care—Will It Survive?" Clearly, major medical organizations are concerned about the exodus of doctors from primary care medicine.

The statistics documenting the trend of physicians away from primary care medicine are convincing. In the last eight years, the number of U.S. graduates entering family practice residencies has dropped by 50 percent. Just seven years ago, half of all internal medicine residents were choosing primary care as a career; currently, only 20 percent of internal medicine residents choose to practice primary care medicine. Eighty percent of all internal medicine residents are now becoming subspecialists or hospitalists, doctors who do shift work in a hospital as opposed to caring for their own patients both in and out of the hospital. Furthermore, many residency slots in primary care are going completely unfilled. Of those spots that do fill, many are being occupied by foreign medical school graduates.

It is clear that if primary care medicine is not reshaped to become a more rewarding and attractive profession, there will be even fewer Dr. Welbys in the future. If this happens, medical care will become even more fragmented. As body parts are parceled out to various subspecialists, there will be no one in charge of the whole patient, no one to coordinate treatment, no one to care about the patient as a person. As a result, patients of all ages will suffer.

THE UNATTRACTIVENESS OF PRIMARY CARE

In addition to the loss of physician autonomy in the new medical order, there are many reasons that primary care medicine has become unappealing to young doctors. Financially, a subspecialist can make about three times the amount of money that a primary care doctor can make, simply by doing expensive procedures. Given that medical school debts range from $100,000 to $250,000, financial pressures to repay educational debt have become a very real factor for young doctors when choosing a career. One consequence of this for patients is that some of the best and brightest of medical students will never even consider a career as a primary care physician.

With the information explosion in medicine, the scope of primary care medicine has become large and difficult to manage. For many medical students, the breadth and depth of knowledge required to effectively practice internal medicine, family medicine, or pediatrics is intimidating. What was known about medical illnesses and their treatments in 1970 is a fraction of what is known today. It is a daunting task for a young doctor to commit to a lifelong study of the full spectrum of medicine. It is also no easy task for practicing primary care doctors to keep up with their continuing medical education. For many young doctors, it just feels more comfortable to become an expert in a small area of medicine and limit the scope of responsibility.

Finally, and perhaps most importantly, there is inadequate time in our current third-party payer model for primary care doctors to practice their craft and spend time with their patients. There is less time to think. There is less time to care. There isn't enough time to delve into complex problem solving. Practicing good medicine under stringent time constraints becomes an impossible task and instead turns into a game of rotating neglect. According to the *New England Journal* article referenced above, it would take a primary care doctor 18 hours per workday to deliver all of the necessary care to his chronically ill patients and the preventative care needed for a panel averaging 2,500 human beings. Nobody can or should consider working this much.

THE DOCTOR–PATIENT RELATIONSHIP AND THE NEEDS OF THE PATIENT

If you were stuck on a desert island and had to choose between being accompanied by a competent doctor or a compassionate but less competent doctor, you'd take the competent doctor every time. However, if you have ever been a patient with a chronic illness, or have ever seen a family member or friend facing a medical crisis, you know that caring is a very important factor in the healing equation.

Especially when dealing with chronic medical illness, the patient has a palpable need to know that the doctor has a genuine interest in him or her as a person. I use the word palpable because as a physician, this need can easily be felt when you look into the eyes of a patient. When the patient visits the doctor, she can sense if the doctor is fully present. Do I have the doctor's full attention? Is he distracted or thinking about something else? Does he really care? Does he know why staying alive is so important to me and what I have to live for?

During my first year of medical school, I distinctly remember a lecture by Dr. Richard Roberts, one of the icons of infectious diseases at Cornell, on the importance of caring. It was not a touchy-feely lecture. It was a talk on bacterial infections. But before talking about bugs and drugs, Dr. Roberts said, "You've all been through a rigorous selection process. Approximately five thousand bright and talented premedical students applied to Cornell for the hundred places you now occupy. However, we know from previous studies and experience that not all of you will become good doctors. To be a good doctor, it takes more than being bright. *You have to like people*. If you don't like people, you'll never be a good doctor."

THE MEDICAL ECOSYSTEM

In a cynical society that often speaks of physician motives in purely mercenary terms, it is important to realize what drives doctors' behavior. Most doctors who enter the field of primary care medicine really do like people. Their motivation goes far beyond financial success. They have important personal and professional needs that are met by meaningful doctor–patient relationships. What happens between a doctor and a patient could accurately be characterized as a symbiotic relationship.

Most primary care doctors have a strong desire to be effective and be of value to other human beings. It is part of their psychological profile. They get something very important from this doctor–patient exchange. It brings meaning to their lives. It also translates to the patient as something of paramount value: the feeling of being genuinely cared for by the doctor.

Few internists or family practitioners have delusions that they will become rich from their calling. Had they wanted to generate cash quickly, they could have opted to run fiber-optic scopes up people's butts twenty times every morning on their way to the bank. I do not say this to disparage my gastroenterology colleagues. Their expertise is critical to the treatment of patients and many are caring, compassionate doctors. But from a personal point of view, it just wouldn't be worth the extra money to me to limit my view of medicine to the insides of people's colons.

So you see, the doctor–patient relationship is not only important for the survival of the patient. It is important to the psychological survival of the doctor. Both species need this interaction. In fact, the quality of this relationship is important to the survival of the entire medical ecosystem. The voracious parasites that have been recently introduced into this environment have caused a severe imbalance in the system. The survival of all of the inhabitants is now threatened.

DR. WELBY ON LIFE SUPPORT

Despite the rumors of Dr. Welby's untimely death, I am happy to inform you that he is still alive and well. Dr. Welby was not murdered. He has merely been on life support. He has suffered many injuries in our current medical system. However, he was not killed during his collisions with HMO executives. He survived his frivolous malpractice suits, although he feels constrained by the need to practice more defensive medicine. He was not suffocated by piles of paperwork from the Medicare bureaucracy. The spirit of Dr. Welby is making a comeback, stronger than ever, in a new practice model that you will learn about in this book.

Since the time of Hippocrates (ca. 460 B.C.), the doctor–patient relationship has faced many challenges. Today's financial threats to this relationship are merely bumps in the road. There will be new threats to the doctor–patient relationship in the future. However, doctors—as intelligent, resourceful, and independent people—will always find ways to re-create environments in which they can properly care for their patients.

In this book, you will read about a movement by competent and caring private doctors who are taking back their profession for themselves and their patients. They are regaining control over the quality of the medicine they deliver. They disagree with the third-party payers who believe patients can be cared for in brief 8- to 12-minute office encounters. They are taking time with their patients. They are establishing a new level of excellence in primary care medicine.

This new breed of doctors is also using evidence-based medicine to show patients how to become healthier and live longer lives than would have ever been possible in Welby's generation. Doctors have new and important information to share with patients on how to make those years more enjoyable and rewarding. Educating and counseling patients about lifestyle changes takes time, but it yields huge returns. Concierge doctors are making time to do this.

Dr. Marcus Welby is back, not as an old codger or a throwback to olden days, but as a caring personal physician who also takes advantage of all the modern technologies of cutting-edge medicine without sacrificing the personal involvement so vital to patients' health and peace of mind. Concierge medicine represents a movement by professionals who recognize the simple truth that caring for patients takes *time*—a tonic which has no substitute and which carries no risk of harmful side effects.

CHAPTER 2

What Is Concierge Medicine and How Does It Work?

Concierge medicine, boutique medicine, and retainer medicine are all terms used to describe a new form of medical phenomenon that is sweeping the country. The topic has been covered on the front page of *The New York Times*, in *Newsweek* magazine and in other national publications. Concierge medicine is a form of private medical care in which patients pay a physician directly for increased time and access to that doctor.

In return for payment, the patient receives services such as guaranteed same-day appointments, 24/7 access to the physician by cell phone or beeper, house calls, emergency room visits, and hospitalizations directed by the private physician. In addition, wellness care and preventative care are often provided. A comprehensive approach to healthcare allows time to address the unique needs of the individual.

What is central to all forms of concierge medicine is that third-party reimbursement to the doctor is either eliminated or relegated to partial payment for the doctor's services. Patients take responsibility for payment. They decide to make a personal investment in their own healthcare.

In practice, concierge medicine is not a single entity. It is a term used to describe many different private financial arrangements between doctors and patients. What all forms of concierge practice have in common is that they represent a return to the privatization of medicine.

WHAT'S IN A NAME?

For critics, the term "concierge medicine" provides the opportunity to paint an image of mercenary doctors at the beck and call of the rich. Senator Pete Stark told the Congress, "Concierge care is like a new country club for the rich." The term smacks of exclusivity. I received this kind of criticism when I opened the first concierge medical practice in the state of Arizona seven years ago. In a caption next to my picture on the front page of the *Arizona Daily Star* was a quote from a University of Arizona medical professor which read, "This is boutique medicine at its mercenary worst."

However, many forms of concierge medicine are now affordable to the middle class. For the cost of a package of cigarettes per day, many people can buy increased time and access to a competent doctor. As I will explain in Chapter 10, there are ways to make concierge medicine affordable to most middle-class Americans.

Because the term has become politically charged, many doctors who practice concierge medicine have abandoned it completely. The first group of concierge physicians to formally organize changed their name from *The American Society of Concierge Physicians* to *The Society for Innovative Medical Practice Design* (SIMPD). According to Dr. Chris Ewin, current President of SIMPD, "the new term is called 'direct practices,' because we have a direct financial relationship with our patients."

Though the term concierge medicine is new to the American vocabulary, private medical practices of this kind have been around for decades. The fees of the Fifth Avenue physicians in New York City have never been paid by insurance companies, HMOs, or Medicare. Wealthy people with means have always paid higher fees for greater medical access and service. In times past, this was done quietly by a few. Having a personal physician is now becoming available to the masses.

Personally, I like the term concierge medicine. Not because it is an accurate reflection of the practice, as it is not. I like the term because it stimulates an honest debate about the need to reform healthcare in America. It causes all of us to decide what we value and what we are willing to pay for. It forces us to look at ethical issues and confront the shortcomings of our current healthcare system. Most importantly, discussions on how we spend our dollar on medical care puts focus on the fact that people should view their health as a *precious asset* that requires a personal investment.

A BRIEF HISTORY OF CONCIERGE MEDICINE

The concierge medicine movement had its beginnings in Seattle, Washington. The concept has been called the brainchild of one of the former physicians of the Seattle Supersonics basketball franchise. The founders of the first concierge practice, called MD Squared (MD^2), were Dr. Howard Maron and his partner, Dr. Scott Hall. MD^2 has been called the platinum standard of concierge care.

MD^2 was opened in 1996. Just like Starbucks, which also originated in Seattle, people with the money could purchase luxury medical care along with "the best cup of coffee in the world." Immediate medical access, which was previously available only to professional athletes, could be purchased for the right price. According to published articles on its Web site, the annual concierge fee for an MD^2 patient is $13,200. A spouse can be added for an additional $6,800, and a child over the age of fourteen can be added for an additional $2,000 per year.

On its Web site, MD^2 states, "There are many concierge practices popping up across the country. MD^2 remains in a class all its own. How? We hand select the most distinguished and accomplished doctors to care for a maximum of fifty families at each of our state-of-the-art clinics. We shepherd each family's health and wellness by providing absolute, unlimited access to their personal physician–a physician who intimately knows their history, their lifestyle, and who can anticipate their needs." When you read statements like these, it is easy to understand why this subject has been characterized in the media as "elitist." However, this is simply part of MD^2's marketing strategy. It is their brand and a description of their exclusive service. It is no different than the advertising strategy of Lexus. They sell a service to wealthy people. I see nothing wrong with this. Over 20 percent of Americans make a bad investment decision every day by getting up and putting a cigarette in their mouths. This behavior costs the country billions in healthcare expenses. If people want to invest $13,000 per year in protecting and improving their health, good for them. It is a wonderful example of good priorities. However, it is very important to realize that MD^2 is only one expensive form of concierge medicine.

When I opened my concierge practice in the year 2000, the concierge movement was still in its infancy. There were only a handful of such practices across the country. Today, it is estimated that there are at least 500 concierge practices in the United States. The numbers are growing every week. The number of physicians who have informal direct financial arrangements with their patients is probably much larger.

TWO BASIC FLAVORS

For the purposes of understanding the concept, I will say that concierge medicine comes in two basic flavors. The first I will call the MD^2 model. In this model, patients pay the entire doctor's fee on their own. It is relatively expensive. Insurance companies are not billed. Medicare is not billed. The patient bears the entire expense of doctor's visits and services in an annual retainer fee. In addition, the patient carries private healthcare insurance. Again, MD^2 doctors limit their practices to a very small number of patients and care for no more than fifty families.

The second model is the MDVIP model. MDVIP is a brand of concierge medicine that was started in Boca Raton, Florida. In this model, patients pay a lower yearly fee of between $1,500 and $1,800 per year. Doctors under this model continue to bill Medicare and private insurance companies as part of the doctor's fee. In programs such as this, the retainer can often be spread out monthly and is only a supplement for those services that are not paid for by Medicare or private insurance.

Doctors in the MDVIP model typically carry much larger panels of patients than the physicians in MD^2. MDVIP doctors may carry up to 600 patients. To put this into perspective, the average internist in this country has 2,500 to 3,000 patients. Even doctors in an MDVIP model have far more time to spend with their patients than those under traditional care.

Both MDVIP and MD^2 have franchised. However MDVIP is by far the larger corporation, operating in nineteen states plus the District of Columbia. MDVIP offers doctors with existing medical practices a turnkey approach to converting their practices to concierge medicine. It is not cheap. According to *The New York Times*, MDVIP charges the doctor a management fee of $500 per patient per year to be part of this franchise, for which it provides legal advice, marketing help, and other business support. *The Times* reported that as of October 2005, nationwide about 250 medical practices and 100,000 patients have signed up for MDVIP and similar corporations.

Which model is better? There are pros and cons to each. The fees are higher in MD^2-style practices, but so is the access and number of services offered. It is largely a personal choice and a matter of what you can afford. Obviously, not everyone can afford MD^2-style services.

MY PRACTICE MODEL

I have created a hybrid model of my own, which is a variation on the MD^2 theme. Since I believe there is great value in being financially and professionally independent, I do not accept Medicare dollars. I do not bill insurance companies or third-party payers when I see concierge patients. I accept a retainer fee as full payment for my services.

Concierge patients on my program pay an annual retainer of $6,000 per year for an individual and $10,000 for a couple. I specialize in complicated medical cases. I like a medical challenge. Some of my sickest patients are seen on a weekly basis. I am in contact through the phone with some of my patients several times a week. However, in my practice, I still carry a group of patients who have been with me for many years. These patients have private insurance. They are not on my concierge plan. Similarly, I see a fair number of chronically ill indigent patients, who pay me nothing for my services.

The reasons for my seeing non-concierge patients are multiple. First, I enjoy providing excellent care to patients who badly need it and cannot afford my services. It gives me satisfaction. Second, I want to keep my skills sharp. I need to see a significant number of patients with varying disease processes. If I took care of only fifty or one hundred wealthy patients, I would be concerned about losing my professional edge. My skills might atrophy. I could find myself parceling out body parts to specialists and being little more than a portal to the healthcare system. I have made a huge investment in my medical career. For me, there has to be a balance in practicing concierge medicine. I want to see enough patients to keep my skills sharp, but not so many patients that I am back on the medical treadmill. I also want to fulfill a personal obligation that I feel to use my skills for those in need. As I've said, concierge medicine is *not* one form of practice but a variety of practice styles that involve a direct financial relationship between the doctor and the patient. Doctors have to decide what practice styles they are most comfortable with, and there is room for differing opinions. Different and creative options provide greater choices for patients.

MY CONCIERGE MENU OF SERVICES

In my practice, patients sign a yearly contract for a list of services that are far from traditional. In addition to receiving a high level of medical care, my patients can avail themselves of state-of-the-art wellness care. These services include the following:

1. Guaranteed same-day appointments for any medical problem. These visits typically last 20 to 30 minutes, depending on the complexity of the problem.
2. No long waits in the waiting room.
3. Twenty-four hours per day, seven days per week phone access to me via beeper or cell phone. I always return my pages within 15 minutes. I answer pages from anywhere on the globe. Many of my patients travel abroad. When they experience a medical problem in London, they will call me for advice.
4. Emergency room visits are supervised by me. I live and practice close to the hospital. I will see a patient in the ER within 30 minutes of an emergency page.
5. I offer comprehensive executive physicals, including sophisticated exercise stress testing not offered by other internists or cardiologists.
6. I offer an in-depth health and fitness consultation. At the end of these consultations, the patients leave with personalized fitness and nutritional plans crafted to meet their specific needs. The plans are tailored to their tastes and goals.
7. I make prompt referrals to leading local and national specialists. In complex cases, I will consult with some of the world's leading medical authorities by phone. I will accompany a seriously ill patient to see a specialist—even if it means boarding a jet and flying with my patient to another part of the country.
8. Patients come to my office for their blood draws, instead of waiting in busy reference labs.
9. I offer a complimentary consultation with a registered dietician and two sessions with a certified personal trainer to help people get started with their health investments. I have a personal training studio in my office with a full gym, so that patients with serious health problems can exercise under direct medical supervision. Should they develop chest pain or other problems while exercising, I am there.

All of these services are included in my annual fee.

WHATEVER IT TAKES

Sometimes my patients need an unusual level of care. Eighteen months ago, an eighty-year-old, robust patient of mine developed a

small tumor in his lung. I had a lung biopsy performed. The pathologists could not determine what kind of tumor he had.

The slides were sent to the senior pathologists at the University of
Arizona. A diagnosis still could not be made. I did some research and
found one of the world's leading pathologists, Dr. Harry Evans, at
the MD Anderson Cancer Center in Houston, Texas. My patient was
diagnosed with a rare, nonpigmented melanoma.

There was no one with much local experience in treating this rare
tumor. I located a world-class melanoma expert at MD Anderson, Dr.
Wen-Jen Hwu. However, my patient did not want to simply turn his
care over to an expert in Texas. This was a difficult problem, and he had
many additional medical problems. He wanted me to hear the advice
of the specialist firsthand. He wanted me to be at his side, interpreting
the information for him during his consultation.

We boarded a private jet and flew to Houston. I accompanied my
patient to the consultation and we flew back. Dr. Hwu set the course of
treatment. I handled the details in Tucson. I found a local oncologist,
Dr. Donald Brooks, who agreed to work with us. When my patient
became short of breath six months later, I diagnosed and treated a rare
drug reaction due to his chemotherapy. I was in contact with Dr. Hwu
and Dr. Brooks. We worked as a team.

The point of the story is not that I get on private jets every day
with my patients—I do not. However, in this case, this is what it took
to find the answer. Could my patient have flown to the Dana Farber
Cancer Institute in Boston and spent a week there getting an oncologist
and a diagnosis? Sure. But this was not what he wanted. He wanted
guidance. He wanted to be an active participant in his care. He wanted
the assistance and judgment of his own doctor to help him sort through
his difficult choices.

In another case, an indigent patient was referred to me from a free
clinic in Tucson. The patient was losing a lot of weight. The clinic doctor was overwhelmed. They asked for my help. I found that the patient
had liver cancer from years of heavy drinking and hepatitis C. This man
could not afford to fly to Texas. However, I found an excellent oncologist in Tucson who was willing to see the patient pro bono. I managed
this patient with the specialist. At the end of his life, I found a hospice
that cared for him free of charge. The man was appreciative of his care.
I had the time in my practice to help him. He was a craftsman and told
me that he wanted to pay for his visits by making me a clock. Though
I wanted no payment, I understood that this was important to him.

The point here is not that I am a nice guy. I am not trying to get Brownie points by taking care of a few indigent patients. The point is that caring for patients takes time. If doctors are liberated from seeing thirty patients a day just to pay for their overhead, they can also do good work in the community.

WHAT IS NOT COVERED IN A RETAINER FEE?

It is important to realize that the retainer fee is strictly a payment for the services of the concierge internist or family practitioner. What you are paying for is the diagnostic skills, the time, and the expertise of the doctor. In addition, you are paying this professional to be your healthcare consultant. This doctor is your medical quarterback and team leader. He directs all the other players on the field.

Obviously, there are many other costs associated with medical care. People often ask, "What about the payment for labs? What about paying for CT scans and specialists? Do I need insurance?"

The answer to the last question is an emphatic yes. People under the age of sixty-five should maintain at least a catastrophic health insurance plan, if not traditional insurance. Those over sixty-five are covered by Medicare for these expenses. Traditional insurance and Medicare cover hospitalizations, surgeries, and other diagnostic tests. The most expensive part of healthcare is often these ancillary services. This is why concierge medicine is not a replacement for insurance. Concierge doctors are not insurance companies. In Chapter 10, I will discuss how to make concierge medicine more affordable using strategies like a health savings account.

I like to think of the concierge fee as "assurance" as opposed to insurance. Insurance involves entering a risk pool that will cover your financial expenses if you have an unforeseen disaster. Assurance is the real security that comes from knowing the doctor who will be answering the telephone at 2 o'clock in the morning if you become ill.

WHAT IS IT WORTH TO YOU?

In summary, concierge medicine is a form of medical practice where a doctor reduces the size of his practice to spend more time with his patients. He offers comprehensive health services that are not included in traditional care. The intent is not only to treat disease, but to maximize the health of his patients. In exchange for this increased time with the physician, the patient uses his own money to pay for the doctor's time. There are many models of concierge care. But the unifying concept is simple. It is a return to privatization, where the patient takes personal responsibility for his health and well-being.

Enrolling in a concierge plan is not a frivolity. It is an investment. It is an investment in the only vehicle that you will ever drive on this planet. If making this kind of investment in your health sounds intriguing to you, read on. In the next chapter, I will explain the *real* reasons to consider concierge medicine. What I have described thus far are merely the features of concierge medicine. I will now discuss the benefits.

CHAPTER 3

The Benefits of Concierge Medicine

What are the benefits of concierge medicine? How does it differ from standard care?

The major benefit of concierge medicine can be summed up in a single and powerful word: *Time*. Time is the currency of excellence. A lack of time requires shortcuts. It breeds mediocrity. There is no substitute for time if medical excellence is the goal.

Concierge medicine allows a doctor to structure his practice so that he has time to spend with his patients. He has time to practice good medicine. The patient has time to actually talk to the doctor. This is not about hand-holding for the rich. This is not about treating the walking wounded. This is about creating the time to practice comprehensive care. To create time, a conventional medical practice has to be retooled.

Given this wonderful luxury of time, the doctor and patient can actually work together to solve problems. Most doctors who practice concierge medicine have practiced conventional medicine for years. They know what it is like to rush from patient to patient. They've had that sinking feeling that comes from knowing that they could have done a better job if they only had more time.

With time, a doctor can also teach a patient to invest wisely in their health. He can help his patients to develop a wellness strategy that reduces disease and achieves optimal health. He has time to act as a patient's advocate, as opposed to having foot soldiers to try to catch what falls between the cracks. Even when a chronic disease can only be managed as opposed to being cured, the doctor and patient can work together to make the best of a challenging situation.

One of the most important tools of healing is something called the *doctor–patient relationship*. In the doctor–patient relationship—as in all important human relationships—rushing can be sensed. You cannot spend 10 minutes of "quality time" with a patient, anymore than you can schedule 10 minutes of quality time with your child after working 14 hours at the office. Starting an egg timer when the doctor walks into the room is no way to practice quality medicine. It is no way to build a therapeutic relationship.

THE IMPORTANCE OF TIME IN DIAGNOSIS

As an internist, I will tell you that 90 percent of all diagnoses are made by taking a careful history. There is no way to shortcut this process. To take a careful history, you actually have to listen to the patient. You have to let the patient talk. To do otherwise is wasteful and inefficient. It is also dehumanizing to the patient.

In my previous professional life, I can't tell you how many times I would walk into an emergency room to find that a patient had spent only a few seconds with the ER doctor. Such ER patients were often tested from stem to stern without having ever spoken more than a few words to a physician. These patients had CT scans, EKGs, blood work, and MRI scans. When I would spend 5 minutes just listening to the patients, they would tell me the diagnosis with their symptoms. Most of the expensive tests were completely unnecessary. Most diagnoses are not made in the CT scanner. Most diagnoses are made with the mind of the doctor. The role of tests is to *confirm* or *rule out* a clinical diagnosis.

There is also no substitute for performing a thorough physical exam. The physical exam is becoming a lost art in medicine. As time pressures increase, the exam is given short shrift. I recently saw a patient for the first time in my concierge program that had been seen by another internist as well as a cardiologist for shortness of breath. This busy internist has an excellent reputation. The patient ultimately had a cardiac catheterization. It was determined that the patient had coronary artery disease. He was started on some medications, but was still short of breath. During my physical exam, I examined the patient with a simple stethoscope. The patient had a loud heart murmur, which was the obvious cause for his persistent shortness of breath. The patient had a critical narrowing of his aortic valve, called aortic stenosis. Why was this simple diagnosis missed?

I know this patient's internist and cardiologist. The internist has an Ivy League training. However, he runs a high-volume practice. The cardiologist is also well schooled. When I looked back at the medical records, both of these doctors had written, "No murmurs are appreciated" in their progress notes. Both of these well-trained doctors would have heard the murmur had they actually put a stethoscope to the chest. What happened? They are not bad doctors. The problem was simply a lack of time. They cut corners and never did a thorough exam.

If this were an unusual story, I would not bother sharing it with you. It is not unusual. I served as Chief of Medicine at a 400-bed hospital and heard these stories every week. I do not tell this story to be self-serving or to criticize my colleagues. Time pressures are probably responsible for more errors in medicine than any lack of clinical skills or training. When a busy doctor is faced with a patient who has five or six active medical problems, how is he to address these problems in a 12-minute office visit? Imagine a doctor stringing twenty or thirty of these complex patients together in a day, each scheduled in a 15-minute slot. Now add to this the fact that 30 percent of those complex patients also have psychological or social issues. The emotional and intellectual toll on physicians is huge. When doctors burn out, it is because they have no more to give. This is a systems problem.

MAKING TIME FOR WELLNESS

Concierge medicine is not just about providing more thoughtful medical care. It is also about wellness. Creating wellness is a priority for many concierge doctors. It is a particular focus of my practice, as you will read in subsequent chapters. Achieving optimal health is as important as dealing with serious illness. What we now know about the benefits of even moderate exercise is astounding. Yet 24 percent of Americans still remain sedentary. Many of my patients are sedentary. They get no exercise at all. People need time to understand why this issue is so important.

In addition to a lack of exercise, many patients have problems with their weight. It is no secret that 61 percent of the population is either overweight or obese. It takes time to help people deal with the problem of excess body fat. There is a lot of bad information out there on how to lose weight. People don't know where to begin.

People have many legitimate questions about weight loss. Most people have busy lives. They have not found an efficient way to integrate exercise and healthy eating into their lives. Without this critical investment in their health, they will dramatically increase their risk of suffering from chronic diseases like heart disease, diabetes, and many cancers. Some sound, well-tailored advice from a trusted doctor can be that ounce of prevention that is worth a pound of cure.

The creation of wellness is a very different process than diagnosing and treating disease. People do not become well by taking supplements or pills. They do not become well by ingesting expensive, designer vitamins. They don't lose weight by following a fad diet, like the Atkins diet, the Zone diet, or the blood type diet. They do not become fit by reading *Five Minutes to Fitness*. What is needed is education, guidance, and a personalized approach—tailored to the individual.

Since exercise is so important to health and vitality, I offer a sophisticated exercise consultation to all of my concierge patients. This process generally takes about an hour. This exercise consultation is in addition to, and separate from, their annual executive physical exam. The process of changing behavior patterns requires follow-up. I ask each of my patients to set personal goals. I assess their initial level of health and fitness. I write a plan to help them efficiently reach their goals. I offer two complimentary sessions with a qualified personal trainer in my office to get them started on the right foot. Interestingly, some of the patients who hated exercise in the beginning discover that the investment really pays off! It helps them feel better.

For patients with weight problems, I ask them to keep a three-day diet log. They bring this food record to their exercise consultation. We review the diet and identify areas of weakness. Where necessary, I will refer them to a registered dietician. To do this kind of work costs money. It takes effort on the part of the patient. It requires time on the doctor's part. Medicare and private insurance companies cannot be expected to pay for wellness care. I don't believe that society *should* pay for this service. Wellness is a personal responsibility. Our medical system is already on its way to bankruptcy. Wellness must be an investment of time and money that is made by the individual.

DOCTOR AVAILABILITY

In addition to more time with the doctor, concierge medicine provides the important benefit of immediate availability. So how does this

24/7 thing really work? Is there really a doctor available every minute, every day for emergency calls? To understand the value of timely access, let me illustrate with an experience of one of my patients.

Mitzi Thomas is one of my favorite patients. She and her husband joined my concierge practice five years ago. Mitzi's husband, Harold, said, "We'll see you every year for our annual physicals. We have a good doctor back in Cincinnati. We'll call you for any medical problems that might arise in Tucson. However, I hope we never really need your 24/7 care. I'd rather pay you every year and never call you."

As fate would have it, I got a page from Harold last year at about 8 o'clock on a Tuesday night. He said that Mitzi didn't want him to call. She bent down to get something from under her desk when she experienced the sudden onset of a severe headache. She took a couple of Advils but wasn't really feeling herself. She insisted that Harold not bother me. He picked up the phone and paged me directly.

I told Harold to put Mitzi in an ambulance. I met her in the ER. Based on the story, I suspected that Mitzi's headache was due to an aneurysm in her brain. Her story was classic. Time was of the essence. Because many people with a ruptured aneurysm have a second, more serious bleed, it is critical that they get immediate medical attention.

As soon as Mitzi hit the ER door, I examined her. I ordered an emergency CT scan of the brain and a sophisticated test called an MR Angiogram. The MR Angiogram outlines the small arteries of the brain. The studies revealed that Mitzi not only had an aneurysm, she also had an unusual anatomy of her cerebral blood vessels.

I contacted an expert in interventional neuroradiology Dr. David Jeck at a hospital on the other side of town that specialized in these problems. Dr. Jeck was able to thread a small catheter into Mitzi's complex anatomy and clot off the aneurysm before it ruptured. Mitzi was in the intensive care unit for several days. Ultimately, she left the hospital with her brain and personality intact. For Harold and Mitzi, concierge medicine was not some "country club for the rich." It was a very sound investment in one of their most precious assets: Mitzi's health.

Imagine what would have happened had Harold not had the availability of a qualified physician to address Mitzi's headache? He may have followed Mitzi's wishes and waited until morning. What if Mitzi had called a busy, traditional practice on the morning after her headache? What if she had been told by a receptionist the next day that she could see the nurse practitioner in a few days or wait to see the doctor in two weeks for her headache? This is an easy diagnosis for any experienced internist. However, when headache symptoms are filtered through an overburdened medical assistant or receptionist, the details can be lost in the story. The information may translate to the doctor as follows:

> Receptionist: "Dr. Brown, Mrs. Smith has a headache. You have thirty patients today. When can we get her in?"
> Dr. Brown: "I can see her in two weeks."

A HEALTHCARE ADVOCATE

The book *Internal Bleeding* addresses the rising frequency of medical mistakes that are made in our overburdened system. The authors state that over 100,000 Americans die each year due to medical mistakes. This is a frightening number.

We all make mistakes, even when we have enough time to do our jobs properly. I've made my own share of mistakes. But when the system is stretched to its limits, mistakes become more plentiful. If you are going to go on a healthcare safari, doesn't it make sense to hire an experienced guide? Wouldn't you like to know where the rhinos and snakes are hiding?

One of the roles of the concierge physician is to act as an advocate for patients. The medical advocate provides several critical functions:

- The concierge physician is the medical decision maker. He analyzes information from specialists. He coordinates care and acts as a captain of the medical ship. He is the repository for all of the patient's medical information. He has the greatest sense of the entire patient. He knows all of the medications the patient is taking.
- The concierge physician is a reliable referral source for specialists. He knows which cardiologist is a wizard with a catheter and which one is distracted by a pending divorce. He knows when to get a second, or even a third, opinion.
- He knows the limits of medical expertise in his community. He knows when and how to go beyond the walls of his own city and find world-class specialists to help solve difficult problems. He has the time and expertise to use medical information effectively.
- He protects the confidentiality of the medical record.
- During hospitalizations, your concierge doctor keeps an eye on your care. He keeps a lookout for common pitfalls in the system. He is available 24/7 to the nurses when they have questions about your care.

- The concierge physician should act as a thorn in your side regarding the scheduling and follow-up of important healthcare screening tests. This includes making sure that you have your colonoscopy, your mammogram, your prostate exam, and your PSA. He does stress testing, not only as a screen for coronary disease, but also as a prognostic tool to assess all causes that put you at a risk of premature death.

Let me give you another illustrative vignette. Henry Sims is a middle-aged man with a family history of prostate cancer. Despite paying his $6,000 annual fee, he was so busy at work that I could not get him into the office for his physical two years ago. I called him on a regular basis to schedule appointments, but he was always too busy to come in. I finally sent him a letter saying, "Forget about the physical. At least come in for your blood work and PSA. We'll do the physical when you have the time."

Henry stopped in for 5 minutes to have his blood drawn on his way to New York. His PSA returned markedly elevated. It had risen over five points in just a year. He had an aggressive, early prostate cancer. He had surgery and was cured of his disease. The investment of paying a medical advocate to stay on top of his routine care had been a good one. Who wants to die of something that is preventable?

In a perfect world, everyone would have a healthcare advocate. Everyone would get these kinds of reminders. However, in our current system in which doctors are carrying thousands of patients, they do not have the time to do this kind of advocacy work. If you invest in a consultant who watches over you, the benefits can be considerable.

IS IT WORTH IT?

So, is concierge medicine really a good investment? Are you beginning to understand the importance of time? It is said that time is money. However, money can also buy you time, in terms of a longer and healthier life, if you choose to invest in your health.

Just a little money can buy time and access to a doctor who can make an important diagnosis. It can buy time for someone to watch over you and advocate on your behalf. It can buy time with a health educator who will teach you in the ways of wellness. If you learn to become stronger and healthier, it may buy you more time on this planet. At a minimum, it will add value to your years. Personally, I can think of no better use of financial capital than to invest it in your health.

CHAPTER 4

The Three Critical Components of Comprehensive Healthcare

The wealthiest man in my concierge practice is a guy named Bob Hansen. Bob is a very wise individual. He is also very practical. I was recently speaking to Bob about investing and growing financial wealth. He said that the guiding principle throughout his entire career of wealth building was *simplicity*. He said, "If the deal is too complicated to explain to me in a few sentences, it's probably not worth doing." This holds whether you're investing millions or a few dollars set aside from each paycheck.

As a doctor, I would say that the same is true of growing your health. There is nothing complicated about it. People who tell you that wellness is complicated are usually trying to sell you something. They will tell you that if you want to lose weight, you must eat their magic combination of foods. If you want to be fit, you have to buy their brand of exercise equipment. If you want a good executive physical, you have to travel to the Mayo Clinic. None of these things is true. Conceptually, improving your health and wellness is not complicated. It is simple.

To achieve optimal health, or what some call wellness, you need only three things: expert medical care; an exercise program appropriate for you; and a sound nutritional plan you can follow for the rest of your life.

I've already told you about the value of having expert medical advice. We are now going to focus on the second and third components. However, I'm not going to just tell you to start jogging and eat broccoli.

I am going to explain the need for exercise and nutrition in a different way than you've ever heard. Using a simple financial analogy, we will explore whether or not your health really *is* an asset. I am going to show you that no matter how wealthy you are, you can't afford to neglect this asset. No matter how much of an intellectual you may be, it is just not smart to be sedentary. Whether you are a man, woman, or child, the same principles apply.

INVESTING IN YOUR HEALTH

Robert Kiyosaki, the best-selling financial author of the book *Rich Dad, Poor Dad*, explains how his rich dad taught him the fundamentals of financial literacy. His rich dad educated him at the age of nine, using simple terms that even a child could understand. Regarding investments, his rich dad said, "The rich buy assets. The poor and middle class buy liabilities that they think are assets."

Kiyosaki goes on to present a simple and elegant explanation of the differences between financial assets and liabilities. Assets are things that put money in your pocket. If you buy assets, they will contribute to a positive cash flow. If you buy liabilities, you will have a negative cash flow. If you want to be rich, invest in assets!

Some examples of assets owned by the rich include securities, rental properties, or businesses. Financial liabilities are things that that masquerade as assets, like fancy homes, cars, and boats. These things are nice luxuries, but they are not assets. They do not put money in your pocket. They do not generate wealth. They consume cash.

Using this simple definition, can you really call your health an asset? Yes, you can! And you should. Your health, your body, and your mind are your most precious assets. They are *not* merely precious possessions—there is an important difference. You need your health to generate wealth if you are to enjoy freedom in your life. You don't believe me? What happens when you are sick and disabled? What happens when a family's primary breadwinner can't work? Or if a single parent has to spend a considerable amount of time off the job? What happens when the CEO of a company has a heart attack or a stroke?

As people examine their balance sheets of life, they do not usually list their health as an asset. Health is often not valued like their Microsoft stock, their bonds, and their businesses. Instead, many ignore their health altogether. Good health is a given. They treat it like a depreciating possession, like some kind of self-cleaning oven that requires no time or maintenance.

However, if you don't presently think of your health as an asset, it may be wise to change your thinking. The dividends that are paid by good health go far beyond financial reward. Good health allows you to enjoy life to its fullest. If you want to enjoy family, friends, hobbies, travel, and even good sex, health is a must. This analogy of health as an asset is not just a play on words. It is not just some cute idea I dreamed up for this book.

If you haven't invested in your health to date, it is not too late. You are not a bad person if you are a late bloomer in this area. I'm not being judgmental here. We all have blind spots. I am simply saying that you need to invest in your health. This means that you have to spend time and money on your health, the way that you invest in other cash-producing assets.

YOUR FIRST CAR

Remember how proud you were when you got your first new car? Do you remember how you took such great care of it? Do you remember how you parked it far from the other cars in the parking lot, so that it wouldn't get scratched? Oh, how you babied that car! You washed it weekly and changed the oil every 3,000 miles.

Even in middle age, many people baby a new car this way. They take the car in for regular tune-ups. Some use only premium gas in their car. If you ask them why they do this, they will look at you incredulously and say, "I paid $70,000 for this car!" However, it is not uncommon to see a middle-aged man get out of his beautiful, new Mercedes 30 pounds overweight and out of shape. By appearance, it is easy to see that he treats his car better than he treats his health.

I have female executives who walk into my office exhausted. Their bone density studies tell me that they are developing osteoporosis; they do no weight bearing exercise. They tell me that they have "no time" to take care of themselves. They are busy growing their businesses and taking care of their families. They fail to take care of the one thing that keeps the whole show going: their health!

DIVIDENDS PAID BY GOOD HEALTH

Good health, by contrast, generates more than dollars. Having good health pays many lifelong dividends. Some of these dividends are even more precious than money.

As long as you continue to invest, good health gives the following return on investment:

- Energy, stamina, and endurance to live your life fully.
- Strength, which can be defined as the ability to resist being captured, damaged, or broken.
- Added years and quality to your years—things you need to enjoy with your spouse, your children, and your family.
- The ability to remain active, engaging in wonderful activities, like traveling, hiking, skiing, or whatever else makes you happy.
- Feeling good inside of your skin. If you radiate health, people are attracted to you. It changes the way that you interact with the world.
- Better sex.
- The ability to enjoy and survive a few decadent pleasures, like the occasional feast or the all-night party. If you are strong and healthy to begin with, you can easily pig out at the office Christmas party or the family reunion without much fallout. We all need the occasional feast! Life should be fun.

WHY DO WE PROTECT AND GROW OUR ASSETS?

If I asked you why you bothered to protect your financial assets—like your business or your investment portfolio—you'd probably look at me like I was crazy. Money, or capital, is hard to come by. Some argue that it is even harder to keep. It is important to protect your wealth. Once you have wealth people want to take it from you. People try to sue you. They slip on your office floor or patio and hope they've won the lottery. The government wants a big piece of your wealth for taxes. What people do to protect their wealth is hire professionals. They hire expensive accountants and lawyers. To anyone with even modest assets, professional fees are absolutely worth the cost. Mistakes cost far more than good professional advice that keeps you out of trouble.

Your health should be protected using the same approach. You need a real healthcare professional as your advocate. Protecting your health asset starts with having a good medical advisor. As I stated earlier, we generate wealth because it buys us freedom. Money buys freedom. Health does the same thing; it buys freedom. Protect your health. Invest in it. While other people may not try to steal your health, the by-products of a sedentary lifestyle can erode your asset. The unexpected infection or injury cannot be prevented. But if you have a reserve of health, you will be better able to tolerate these unpredictable events.

Once you have financial capital, you want to do more than merely protect it. You want your capital to grow. Smart people do not put their money in a mattress. They do not lock their cash in a safe deposit box. With inflation and cost of living increases, the money will be worth less in five years than it is today. You want your money to grow and to work for you. The same should be true of your health!

As I explained in my first book, *The Body-Mind Connection*, there is no such thing as staying the same as far as health is concerned. At any point in time, you are either in the process of getting stronger or getting weaker. You are either making sound health investments, or your health assets are depreciating.

WHAT WELLNESS IS NOT

Wellness has become a wastebasket term that is used very loosely in our culture. It is liberally applied to the sale of many health products and services. The wellness industry is a multibillion-dollar industry. It encompasses everything from the sale of untested supplements and designer vitamins to magnets and aromatherapy. At most high-end spas, a smorgasbord of services is offered under the guise of wellness. If you want a good business, go into wellness! There is a lot of cash to be made.

I have no professional objections to people doing whatever makes them feel good. I get massages myself. It feels good. It relieves stress. If people want to spend their money relaxing with aromatherapy for stress reduction, this may well benefit them. However, if you tell me that you are going to invest in magnets, aromatherapy, and garlic as a way to get healthy, I am skeptical. There is no data that these things will improve your health. If you think these are optimal investments, you may want to reconsider. Most products that are sold for wellness are nothing but illusions.

Feeling well comes from *being* well. You will feel well if you have more lean muscle, less fat, and greater stamina. At its core, *wellness is a performance issue*. The performance of your body can be easily measured. Unless you are willing to invest in improving the way that your body performs, you are not going to have health-wealth.

MEASURING WEALTH

In the world of finances, numbers are used to determine the present value of an asset. Entrepreneurs do not pay the asking price for a piece of real estate without looking at the numbers. If an investor is going to buy a duplex, he wants to know what the property will generate in income. Will this duplex be an asset or a liability? The only way to know is to look at the numbers. As you will see, the same is true of health.

The Story of Bill and Jack

Let's look at two men, Bill and Jack. They both live in an upper-middle-class suburb. They are both forty-eight years old. They each have similar new cars in the driveway. Both send their kids to private schools. From appearances, it looks like Bill and Jack are both doing well financially.

Bill has a seventh grade education. He owns a garbage collection business. He is street-smart. His home is paid for. He has $100,000 per year in passive income from some real estate investments. His Lexus is paid off. He recently sold a piece of property from his dump. He now has a net worth of $2,000,000, which is wisely invested and growing. These are Bill's numbers. They give a clear picture of Bill's financial health.

Jack is a doctor. He just went through a costly divorce. His wife got the big house. Jack had to scale down and moved into Bill's neighborhood. Jack got the bank loan on the couple's boat for $160,000 at an 8 percent interest rate. He fought for the boat in the divorce. He viewed it as an asset. There are expensive docking fees and maintenance charges. Jack has a mortgage on his new home of $500,000. He has $20,000 in credit card debt. Jack has no measurable net worth except for some paper equity in his home. Bill and Jack live in the same neighborhood, but their numbers tell a very different story.

MEASURING HEALTH

Wellness and health can be measured just as financial wealth can be measured. People like Bill and Jack can look similar on the outside, just like their possessions. Without the numbers to accurately assess the facts, looks can be deceiving. Health numbers are also needed to tell an accurate story. Health numbers are very precise. As a doctor who measures health daily, the numbers tell me everything.

If I am making a health assessment for you, I need to know how well your body functions under stress. I need to know how much extra body fat you are carrying. To give you good advice on how to invest, I need to know how much lean muscle you have. What is your bone density? What is your blood pressure? What is your cholesterol? How long can you last on a standard exercise treadmill test? This is objective information that paints an accurate health picture.

Bill and Jack's Health Portfolio

Let's say that Bill and Jack both come to see me for a health assessment. I offer to do two simple health tests to examine their health portfolio. They agree to undergo an exercise stress test and have a body composition test.

An exercise stress test does far more than screen for coronary disease. It gives a doctor an objective measure of your aerobic fitness. The number of minutes you last on a treadmill is one of the most important benchmarks of health. Aerobic fitness is linked to wellness and longevity.

A body composition test, as opposed to your weight, tells a doctor how much extra fat you are carrying. It tells him how much lean, healthy muscle you have. You can get a good approximation of body fat by using a simple handheld device that many doctors have in their offices.

Jack, our recently divorced doctor, is under a lot of stress. He does not exercise regularly. He has not made time to do so in years. I put Jack on the treadmill. He lasts only 7 minutes before telling me that he's had enough. I tell Jack that for a person of his age and sex, he should have lasted at least 9 minutes. So what? What's the big deal about 2 lousy minutes? Is Jack going to die earlier if he is a little less fit than he should be? Maybe. In fact, unless he begins investing in his health, he very well may leave the planet earlier than his friends.

Published studies in the *New England Journal of Medicine* have shown that time on a treadmill is a better predictor of premature cardiac death than any other risk factor for heart disease. People who performed just 15 percent below their expected level of fitness *doubled* their risk of cardiac disease and premature death! This goes for both men and women.

After a stress test like Jack's, I would sit down with him and have a heart-to-heart talk. I'd explain the meaning of low fitness. I would ask Jack to make an investment in his health. If he were just beginning to invest, I might suggest a brisk walking program to start. If he had been previously athletic, I'd find out what he liked to do in the past. We would work together and find some form of exercise that fit into Jack's stressful and busy lifestyle. I would explain to Jack that his current lack of aerobic fitness was a true liability.

Bill, on the other hand, had a much better stress test. Bill exercises daily. He plays soccer on the weekends with his buddies. He performs physical labor at work. Bill lasted 11 minutes on his stress test. In this case, I would have the pleasure of explaining to Bill that he scored 20 percent above what we would expect for his age and sex. I'd tell Bill that from a health perspective, he had the equivalent of money in the bank. Bill has a reserve of health and fitness that will stand him in good stead in the future. If he becomes ill or has an accident, Bill is in a better position to weather the storm.

BODY COMPOSITION

Grace and Sue

A few years ago I gave a talk on women's health to a group of female physicians. After the talk, one of my infectious disease colleagues, Dr. Elizabeth Wack, quipped, "So, what my mother told me was right. You can never be thin enough or rich enough!" Liz was commenting on the data that I had presented regarding body composition and women's health. This issue goes far beyond any superficial discussions of appearance. Body composition in women is a critical issue in assessing their health portfolios.

Let's look at this assessment to get some meaningful numbers. Grace is a forty-year-old woman who has not invested much in her health. Like Jack, she's been "too busy" to exercise. She works hard running her own publishing business. Her business is strong and she has invested her profits wisely. When she leaves the office after a busy day, it's not to spend a relaxing evening at home, but to start the second shift—she's raising two kids. So to save time, Grace frequently stops for dinner at fast-food restaurants. The kids beg her to stop at McDonald's. She ends up eating what they eat. However, Grace doesn't burn the calories that her kids burn. She is sedentary. I measure Grace's body composition. Thirty-three percent of her total weight is made up of body fat. Is this a health liability? Yes it is.

Her friend Sue is within a few pounds of Grace on the scale. However, Sue exercises regularly. She has a personal trainer and has a lot of healthy muscle mass. She doesn't look like a body builder, but she is fit. Sue is only carrying 20 percent body fat. Is this good for Sue? You bet it is! It makes her health portfolio much stronger.

Excess body fat is a true liability for women and men both. This is not an issue of cosmetics or vanity. Increased body fat increases your risk of disease. In women, it increases the risk of breast cancer and ovarian cancer significantly. Women with excess body fat become their own estrogen factories. Excess body fat also increases a woman's risk of diabetes, heart disease and stroke. It increases her risk of depression. Besides, it saps her of energy and makes her feel bad! There is less energy to work and less energy to raise the kids. There is no energy at the end of the day for Grace to have a little fun.

In a *New England Journal of Medicine* study published in 1997, lean women who exercised vigorously 4 hours per week had a relative risk of breast cancer of 0.28. In layman's terms, this means that lean, very active women reduced their risk of breast cancer by 72 percent compared to average women. Even moderate exercise, without the leanness, reduces the risk of breast, ovarian, and colon cancers by about 30 percent. Excess body fat is a liability that can be easily measured. These numbers give me much more information than the number on a scale.

Right or wrong, fair or unfair, nature or nurture, the fact is that most women, in addition to holding jobs, take primary responsibility for the home and family. Usually they do the lion's share of cooking, cleaning, caring for any children, and even planning the family's social life. This puts additional stress on them and their health and makes good healthcare especially crucial. A wise woman invests in her health; a smart man helps her do so.

OTHER HEALTH NUMBERS

When I perform evaluations for patients regarding their health port-folios, I want to know more than their time on a treadmill and body compositions. I use these two measurements only as an example. In my practice, I take a comprehensive look at all of my patients' health parameters. Other important numbers that help paint a more complete picture are as follows:

- Cholesterol measurement
- Blood pressure
- Bone density
- Complete blood count and chemistry profile
- Results of screening tests, such as a mammogram for women, PSA for men, and a colonoscopy where appropriate

These are just a few of the numbers that go into a health valuation. When doing sophisticated health assessments, it is important to have someone who can help you interpret the data. You also need someone to guide you on what tests are useful and what tests are not. For example, some patients ask me about something called a Heart View Scan—a CT scan of the heart that measures calcium deposits in the coronary arteries. Others want to consider a total body CT scan, to detect early cancers. These tests are controversial. They expose you to a small but not insignificant amount of radiation and they may increase the risk that you will develop cancer during your lifetime. Before you pay for these kinds of assessments, you should speak with a trusted medical advisor.

GROWING YOUR HEALTH ASSETS

If we determined that your health assessment is poor, how might you make it better? How could we work together to come up with an investment strategy that would pay you dividends in the future?

As your doctor, I would first help you establish a plan to become fitter. I might work with you developing a good nutrition and weight loss strategy—something that *you* could live with. As a concierge doctor, I have time to do this. I would tailor my advice specifically to you. I would not give Bill and Jack the same exercise program. I would write very different exercise prescriptions for Grace and Sue. Generic health advice regarding exercise and nutrition is no more appropriate than generic financial advice. Advice must be tailored to the starting position and goals of the individual.

I can't emphasize enough the need to individualize a plan for exercise and nutrition! Each one of us has a unique body. We each have a unique medical history. We have different goals. We have different levels of motivation. We have unique time constraints. Some of us like to jog; some can barely climb a flight of stairs. Many people have joint problems, back problems, or other medical issues that need to be factored into the equation. Having a physician who knows your entire medical history and has a sense of you as a person is invaluable in crafting a health program.

If Jack, our unfit doctor, took my advice and invested in his health, what kind of return might he expect? Can I project a return on investment for Jack? The answer comes from an article published in the *Journal of the American Medical Association* written by Dr. Steven Blair of the Cooper Clinic. Over 9,000 men who went to the Cooper Clinic in Dallas were given an initial treadmill test. All of them were given good investment advice and told to go home and exercise. The men were invited back five years later and tested again. Some men took the advice and increased their aerobic assets; some stayed sedentary and did not.

The men who increased their level of fitness had a 44 percent reduction in all-cause mortality compared to men who did not invest in their fitness. This is an extraordinary return on investment! If I guaranteed a return on a *financial* investment of 44 percent by asking you to invest just 30 minutes of your time, three days per week, you'd jump at the chance. If the investment paid off in terms of a longer and healthier life, it might be worth even greater consideration.

If I gave Grace some advice on exercise, such as a walking program, what kind of return might she expect? Numbers from The National Nurses Health Study show that women who exercise just two to four times per week reduce their risk of developing heart disease, the number one killer of women, and type 2 diabetes by 30 percent.

How Much Do I Need to Invest?

The good news is that you will need to invest much less to grow your health than you would to grow your wealth. All of the major studies on exercise have shown that the greatest benefit comes in moving from a sedentary lifestyle to a moderately active lifestyle. By simply walking 3 hours per week, you could dramatically reduce your chances of developing diabetes, suffering from a heart attack, or contracting breast cancer.

In my experience, once people get a taste of the benefits, they want to invest more. The most unlikely of candidates in my practice—people who have been sedentary all of their lives—are often the ones who make the greatest changes.

If you are already pretty healthy and you want to invest further, there are investment strategies for you as well. I have patients in my practice who decide to become fit by training for a marathon. In these cases, I employ state-of-the-art technology to help them reach their goals. This may seem silly to some, but this is what they want. In my practice, the individual drives the investment. It is the concierge physician's role to provide the expertise.

Health Liabilities and What They Do to Your Assets

A liability like excess body fat depreciates your most precious asset. It wears out your hips and your knees prematurely. It clogs up your arteries. It decreases your self-esteem. It dramatically increases your risk of diabetes, which is a systemic disease of small blood vessels. Diabetes is not a disease of sugar. It is a disease of blood vessels. It causes premature heart attacks, strokes, erectile dysfunction, and a host of other maladies.

A lack of fitness can also depreciate your mental health. Sedentary and overweight individuals are at much greater risk of depression. In fact, exercise can even be used as therapy for depression. In a study done at Duke University, sedentary depressed patients were randomly assigned to either a supervised exercise program or the drug Zoloft. After sixteen weeks, the results were identical. In my practice, I certainly do not hesitate to use antidepressants where appropriate. However, I also encourage my depressed patients to help themselves with a little movement.

HOW DO YOU INVEST IN EXERCISE?

Exercise is a dirty word for many people. They don't particularly enjoy it. I have many people in my practice who view exercise like taking castor oil. They "hate it." When I first started doing exercise consultations ten years ago, I would ask my patients, "What exercise do you like the most?" This question worked until I met the first person who responded, "None . . . I hate all exercise." I thought for a moment and said, "Good. What form of exercise do you hate the least?" She smiled and said, "Walking."

When I am dealing with the legitimate dislikes of someone who finds exercise as enjoyable as balancing a checkbook, I focus on efficiency. I develop a plan that will produce the greatest return for the shortest investment of time. Many of my patients are very busy. Their life is a process of multitasking. They need to be efficient. Thirty minutes of well-planned activity three times per week can make a tremendous difference.

After an initial health assessment by your physician, you determine where you are starting from. Next, you will have to determine where you want to be. You need to establish wellness and fitness goals. With a clear goal in mind, you should honestly decide how much time you want to invest in your goals. With these pieces of information, you can go about mapping out a plan with your doctor. If you don't know where you are starting from, where you want to be, and how you are going to get there, you will just get lost.

After you start your program, you will need periodic assessments every three to six months. You won't need a stress test every three months, but you will need to follow some objective parameters at periodic intervals. If your numbers are not improving, you will need to change your investment strategy. I will discuss the details of this process in the next chapter.

Bad Health Investments

Financially strong people like Bill build their wealth before they purchase the fun little liabilities. The fancy stuff, like homes and cars, are not financial hardships when you have the money. They are luxuries or icing on the cake. People without personal wealth, like Jack, buy the icing before they have the cake.

People like Jack often eat the way that they spend money. They consume rich foods because it makes them feel wealthy. However, they are only creating health debt before any level of wellness has been achieved.

When people go out to a fancy restaurant and order two cocktails, a Caesar salad (which contains 50 grams of fat), and a New York strip steak and finish up with crème brûlée, they feel like a rich person. For a few moments, they feel like a king. However, when that illusion of wealth is gone, they are left with health liabilities. Their waistline is bigger. They are more short of breath as they walk up the stairs. They may realize that they have made a bad investment in their health. But they don't change their strategy. This is why more than 60 percent of Americans are either overweight or obese. They eat rich all the time. They don't invest in exercise.

When you continually eat foods that are rich in fat and sugar, you are making bad investments in your health. What you are doing is adding to your liability column, not your asset column. A rich diet creates the liability of excess body fat. It depreciates your most precious asset.

Don't get me wrong; this stuff tastes good. Sure, it's okay to give yourself a treat from time to time. But if you want health, you can't do this all the time. Just as you don't waste your money buying everything that your heart desires, so you would be wise to invest in eating healthier foods.

WHAT IF YOU ALREADY HAVE A CHRONIC ILLNESS?

Is it too late to start exercising if you have serious, chronic medical problems? What if you are "too old" to exercise? Have you missed the window of opportunity?

Absolutely not! I specialize in writing exercise prescriptions for people with complex medical problems. I am now working with Dr. David Alberts, the Director of the University of Arizona Cancer Center, to help young doctors write exercise prescriptions for cancer patients. I have written programs for people with severe emphysema, cancer, coronary artery disease, congestive heart failure, and diabetes. People with chronic illnesses often get the greatest benefits from exercise. The reason is that much of the fatigue that is attributed to their chronic illness is actually due to physical deconditioning. When you are ill and sedentary, your muscles atrophy. You lose aerobic fitness. With a little exercise, you begin to regain your fitness, and you perform much better. You feel less fatigued, at any age.

I have an extraordinary eighty-two-year-old woman in my practice, Marie Hansen, who has had nine separate cancers. She has had breast cancer, endometrial cancer, lung cancer, metastatic melanoma, bladder cancer, and thyroid cancer. She has had a small heart attack. She also has emphysema. Marie did not start exercising until she was seventy-seven years old. She now spends 30 minutes every day on the treadmill. She works out with a personal trainer two times per week. Marie is worth a great deal of money. Now she is investing in her health. At age eighty-two, she understands that this is her most precious asset.

Marie had a lobe of her right lung removed for cancer two years ago. A year later, I repeated her stress test. After investing in her exercise program, she actually lasted longer on her treadmill test than she did *before* her lung surgery! She attributes her exercise program with saving her life. If Marie can get this kind of return on her investment at seventy-seven, you can as well. I have two patients in their nineties who exercise every day. They are vibrant and wonderful women.

SO WHAT SHOULD YOU EAT?

I've told you what not to eat. By now, you may be wondering what I think you should eat. To get you to read this far, I've bent the truth just a little. Actually, I *am* going to suggest that you eat more broccoli. If not broccoli, maybe some other colored vegetables rich in vitamins and antioxidants that you like. Though I'm not suggesting that you become a vegetarian, I would like you to understand the benefits of eating a few more veggies.

If all we cared about were reducing your liability column of fat, I would advise you to eat fewer calories. You could eat 800 calories per day of almost anything and lose body fat. I could put you on an 800 calorie-per-day butter diet and you would lose weight. This is because weight loss is merely a matter of limiting calories. However, there is more to optimal nutrition than calorie balance. What you need in order to invest in your health is *fuel*. You need critical nutrients that help you grow healthy tissue. You need to repair cells damaged by environmental stressors.

It is not enough to get vitamins and nutrients from a vitamin tablet. In fact, there are no good studies to show that expensive or even over-the-counter vitamins make a difference. A recent meta-analysis revealed that patients who took antioxidant supplements actually had a 5 percent increase in mortality compared with those who did not. The data on vitamins is presently not very encouraging, as opposed to the return on investment when you increase the number of nutrients found in whole foods.

In a study published in the *Journal of the American Medical Association* in 1999, an increase in fruits and veggies proved to be a good investment in brain health. This study involved over 75,000 women and 38,000 men. It showed that five to six servings of fruits and veggies per day reduced the risk of stroke by 31 percent. Similarly, the DASH diet, which was published in the *New England Journal of Medicine*, showed that a diet rich in vegetables and nonfat milk products reduced blood pressure. The DASH diet reduced blood pressure to the same degree as using a single medication for hypertension. It accomplished this goal within two weeks. It was effective in men and women and worked in all ethnic groups.

Tailoring Nutrition Advice

Though most experts agree that Americans need more vegetables and lean foods in their diets, this is old news. Just like exercise, nutritional programs need to be *individualized*. It does no good to tell a meat-and-potatoes guy to start dining at his local salad bar. No matter what I say, he is just not going to do it. As doctors, we need to be flexible. We need to be a little more resourceful and versatile in our approach. It is silly to recommend one diet for everyone.

What I do in my concierge practice is to have people start by recording a three-day diet log. I tell them to eat whatever they normally eat. I ask them *not* to change their eating habits just because I will be reviewing their log.

Once I know what someone is really eating, I can begin to suggest some healthy changes. More importantly, once *they* realize what they are eating, we can begin to have an honest conversation. To invest in yourself, you may want to switch from the idea that food is a reward for all of the stress that you have to endure in your life to the idea that food is a fuel for your body. By eating better, you are not depriving yourself of liabilities. You are making an investment in your most precious asset. Again, this is not to say that people cannot have the occasional feast. A life without feasts is just not a rich life. It is just that eating like a king all the time is going to break the health bank.

Most of the behavioral science literature shows that we all make changes slowly. This is true of changes in eating patterns as well. We don't go from eating a bad diet one day to eating a good diet the next. We start limiting bad investments. We often relapse. We learn from our mistakes. We try again. Ultimately, we succeed. In a concierge model, there is time to individualize an approach to diet. There is continuity of care so that improvements in nutrition can be ongoing.

WOMEN AS HEAD OF HOUSEHOLD ON HEALTH

It has been my experience in medicine that women seem to be more interested in making an investment in their health than men. They are more concerned about their own health and that of their family members. Though they may not think in terms of health as an investment, they know that good health must be a priority for a full life.

I have rarely seen a man drag his wife into my office for a visit. Instead, I frequently see a man who is pushed into my office by a concerned wife who recognizes that her husband is ignoring his health. It is usually a mother who calls me about the child with a fever. It is the daughter who brings her aging parents into my office, concerned about their healthcare. Over the past seven years of practicing concierge medicine, I've been called by many wives and daughters of powerful men, asking me to assume the care of their sick husbands or fathers. The father doesn't call me about his medical problems. The daughter calls!

Until more men begin to understand the importance of investing in their health, it will be women who drive improvements in healthcare. One of my patients, a retired nurse and successful businesswoman, has signed up her two adult sons on my concierge plan. It is her desire to instill a proactive attitude toward health in her children. She wants her sons to establish a good relationship with a doctor. She wants them to make time for exercise. She wants them to eat well.

SUMMARY

Following the wisdom of keeping things simple, you need only three critical elements to protect and invest in your health.

1. You will need a good relationship with a doctor to protect your health. You need this in case you get ill. You need a health advisor to help

you learn *how* to get healthier. You need a doctor who takes a proactive approach to detecting problems, before they become acute. This takes time. This is why I suggest you find a concierge physician.

2. You will need to invest in your most precious asset by spending some time on exercise. You will need a plan. You will need some professional support and direction. The return on your investment will be proportional to the time that you put in.

3. You will need a healthy eating plan that you can follow for life; a plan designed by your doctor and individualized to you.

THE CONCIERGE DOCTOR AS TEACHER

If you consult the *Merriam-Webster's Dictionary*, you will see that the first definition of the word doctor is "teacher." The second definition is "one skilled or specializing in the healing arts." The role of the concierge physician is really to help you in both areas.

What you need to achieve optimal health is a health mentor and partner. You need someone who will not talk *at* you, but give you the information and guidance that you will need to *learn* about your own body. When you have that "Aha!" moment about the value of your health, investing in it will not seem like such a chore. It will become fun. When you feel better inside your own skin, the time and money will have been well worth it.

CHAPTER 5

A Day in the Life of a Concierge Physician

INVESTING IN A CONCIERGE DOCTOR

Throughout this book, I have encouraged you to think about your health as an asset. I've suggested that you invest in your health. In managing any personal assets, there are two primary goals: to protect them and to make them grow.

In the upcoming chapters on exercise and nutrition, I will focus on how your concierge doctor can help you grow your health assets. In this chapter, I am going to focus on the doctor's role in protecting them—how your doctor deals with threats from diseases and unforeseen medical problems. To the extent that he has the mechanisms in place to protect you, this goal will be accomplished. To the degree that he is overburdened and overworked, your assets may be more vulnerable.

A HEALTH INVESTMENT ANALYST

Some people are brilliant at managing their own finances. They don't need any financial advice, financial analysts, coaches, or other professionals. However, these people are very rare. Most people need financial consultants—professionals with experience and objectivity who examine an entire financial portfolio to make sure its investments are sound and balanced and suggest adjustments to maximize safety and return.

A concierge physician serves a similar role in analyzing and protecting your entire health portfolio. It is his job to sit back, look at the entire picture, and make sure that all the individual parts of your medical care work together. When you have serious problems, he addresses them promptly and thoroughly.

HOW YOUR HEALTH ANALYST OPERATES

Our current third-party payer system exerts tremendous financial pressures on most doctors to see a large number of patients. An overextended doctor crams as many patients as he can into every available hour. Why? It is simply a question of economics. It has nothing to do with good patient care. Overscheduling can weaken the entire structure of a doctor's medical practice.

From a business perspective, the only commodity the doctor has to sell is his time. He does not sell products that provide him with a source of passive income. He doesn't sell goods like a retailer. To make more money, the doctor must see more patients.

In the current healthcare model, a drop in reimbursement from a third-party payer causes an immediate drop in income from the doctor's business. If Medicare or the HMO lowers its rates, income from the practice drops. If an insurance company or Medicare fails to pay on time, the practice suffers a cash flow crunch.

If the reduction in payment to the doctor resulted in a cost savings to you, at least you would derive some small financial benefit. However, this is not the case. If the doctor's reimbursement rate is cut by 20–50 percent, the "savings" are not passed on to you but are used to pay the administrative fees of the HMO, such as dividends to stockholders and inflated executive salaries. Neither the patient nor the doctor benefits; the only winners are the administrators who ration your time with your doctor.

The key point is that if reimbursement rates fall, the only way the doctor can maintain cash flow is to see more patients. Similarly, if expenses go up, the doctor must see more patients. If malpractice premiums rise, the doctor must see more patients. Though a doctor is held to a higher ethical standard in our culture than a typical businessman, he is still running a business. No matter how kind and devoted he is to his patients, he still has to meet payroll every two weeks.

Doctors are not like employees who get a cost-of-living raise. Doctors' rates do not automatically go up every year. On the contrary, Medicare and other third-party payers have continued to cut reimbursement rates over the last decade. Most doctors' incomes continue to go down. What is even more ominous for doctors in a third-party system is that Medicare is planning to reduce reimbursements even further over the next five years. During this time, malpractice rates and overhead will continue to rise.

Aside from the impersonal experience of dealing with a doctor who is rushed, this situation can be unsafe for patients. The more rushed a doctor is, the more likely he is to make a mistake. While it's fun to watch a juggler put as many balls in the air as he can until one finally drops, you don't want your doctor playing this game with your health. Inadequate time to address medical problems is a factor in medical malpractice. Mistakes made from rushing drive medical malpractice premiums up which causes the price of healthcare to escalate even further, which means doctors must see even more patients.

This vicious cycle of falling reimbursements and rising expenses creates an unsustainable business structure. It has nothing to do with the Hippocratic oath. It is a matter of simple accounting. This untenable business model is responsible for the two problems that bother patients most: shorter visits with the doctor and a plummeting quality of medical care.

Let's take a look at a day in the life of a typical doctor and see how an unstable practice structure affects you, the patient.

Busy Dr. Black

Dr. Black is a primary care doctor. He runs a typical American medical practice. He accepts most third-party payers. He takes private insurance. He accepts HMOs, PPOs (preferred provider organization), and every other kind of O. He accepts Medicare assignment. Most of the insurance companies pay Dr. Black according to Medicare rates. Medicare rates are already discounted well below what Dr. Black has printed on his office price list. However, this doesn't matter. This price list is only what Dr. Black *thinks* he should be paid in an ideal world. He never actually gets paid his established rates. He might as well list $1,000 per visit for his fee instead of $65 per visit. Medicare will only pay him about $55 for a routine 15-minute office visit. "Sorry, Dr. Black, these are the rules."

Under the law, Dr. Black cannot charge his patients any more than what Medicare will allow for each visit. If he sets his rates higher, he cannot ask the patient to make up the difference. He can't charge $65 per visit and ask the patient to pay the extra $10. To do so would be illegal.

Knowing what is driving Dr. Black's assembly-line scheduling practices will help you understand why your current doctor may not have enough time for you, and if you are trying to protect your most precious asset, you need to know what is going on behind the scenes in your doctor's medical practice. Put simply, Dr. Black's cash flow is directly linked to the number of people that he can see in a day and the only way for Dr. Black to see more patients is to give each one just a little less time.

THE ADVENT OF THE "HOSPITALIST"

In addition to time pressures, these third-party forces affect the way Dr. Black practices medicine. He can no longer afford to go to the hospital to care for you when you become seriously ill because to keep his business afloat he's stuck in the office running from exam room to exam room seeing more patients. Dr. Black doesn't like this change. He liked taking care of his patients in the hospital or even at their homes. But it's a matter of economics. He has to pay his staff and his rent.

Is it good for you to have another doctor taking care of you when you are seriously ill in the hospital? Not really. As your doctor, Dr. Black is the one who knows you best. When your care is handed off to another group of unknown doctors in the hospital, called "hospitalists," there will be an inevitable loss in the continuity of your care. It becomes fragmented. One hand does not know what the other is doing. Doctor Black does not know what the hospital doctor is doing. The hospitalist doesn't know what Dr. Black has done for you in the office. There is little or no communication between the two.

Furthermore, there are some not-so-subtle financial pressures from third-party payers to keep Dr. Black out of the hospital. The hospital has its own financial problems. The hospital gets paid a set amount of money for each diagnosis that a patient carries, based upon something called a DRG or diagnostic related group. The hospital does not get paid for a sick person by the day, like a hotel, but by the specific medical problem, independent of how long it takes to treat that problem. Therefore, the hospital likes to employ its own hospital doctors to keep pressure on them to be "efficient"—in other words, to limit treatment to the ethical minimum.

DRGs have changed the way that many doctors behave. Just yesterday, I was called by a hospitalist and asked to see a patient who was being discharged after complications from alcoholism. I was on call for the hospital for patients who did not have a doctor that day. The hospitalist said, "My only concern is his blood pressure elevation." When I asked a few questions, it became clear that the patient was experiencing blood pressure problems from acute alcohol withdrawal. His last drink had only been 48 hours earlier. I asked the hospitalist if it wouldn't be wise to keep him in until he was stable. The hospitalist immediately agreed and changed his plans. This is how financial pressures can influence the judgment of doctors. This hospitalist knew what he should do. He understood medicine. However, in the hierarchy of his thought patterns, his medical judgment was overridden by financial pressures from his employer.

Hospitals and HMOs prefer to use hospitalists. Hospitalists are under the hospital administration's scrutiny. The administration can put pressure on the hospitalists to get people out of the hospital as early as possible. This way, the hospital can make more money on each patient. Do you begin to see how these financial pressures might affect the protection of your precious health assets, especially when you need protection the most?

Dr. Black's Scheduling Structure

Dr. Black schedules patients every 15 minutes—hour after hour, day after day. Sometimes he will even schedule patients every 12 minutes and see five patients in an hour.

This is what Dr. Black's schedule looks like:

8:00	John Green	10:00	Samuel Farmer
8:15	Betsy Strand	10:15	Gene Stamper
8:30	Jim Wesley	10:30	Sandra Chow
8:45	Stan Shine	10:45	Scott Welsh
9:00	Sheryl Smith	11:00	Jennifer Bliss
9:15	Millie Christenson	11:15	Terrence Shilling
9:30	Ben Whittle	11:30	Wilma Franz
9:45	Miriam West	11:45	Tim Chance

Accountants and lawyers don't schedule their time in this way. I know of no other professionals who work like this. This kind of scheduling is even more irrational when you consider the need for the human touch in the practice of medicine.

Dr. Black begins his office hours at 8 A.M. By noon, he has already seen seventeen patients—sixteen scheduled plus one walk-in. Today, his staff has scheduled a "free lunch" provided by a drug representative. Dr. Black doesn't like drug reps. He knows that he shouldn't be getting his prescribing information from them, but he doesn't have much time to read anymore. He is seeing too many patients to keep up. He wolfs down a dry turkey sandwich as the drug rep presents a canned talk about why Drug X is better than the competition. Dr. Black is tired. As he pretends to listen to the salesman's propaganda, he is already thinking about his busy afternoon. From 1 P.M. to 5 P.M. his schedule will be a repeat of the morning's difficult grind.

Dr. Black strategically slips out of the drug talk, pretending to answer his pager. At least he's gotten a free lunch. He signs for his free drug samples and goes back into his office. He looks at the picture of his family on his desk. He feels like his time is slipping away from him. He's missed a lot of soccer games over the years, and for what? This grueling schedule? By the end of his unhappy day, he has seen over thirty patients. He is exhausted. None of his patients got much of his time. In fact, the system makes it impossible. According to the *New England Journal of Medicine*, "It would take 10.6 hours per working day to deliver all recommended care for patients with chronic conditions, plus 7.4 hours per day to provide evidence-based preventive care, to an average panel of 2500 patients." Since docs can't work 18 hours per day to give patients what they need, things fall through the cracks. This is not why Dr. Black went into medicine.

This schedule is not only stressful, but also mind-numbing. Trust me. I've done it. I've practiced like Dr. Black. This is not some construct of my imagination. Thousands of doctors practice like this every day.

THE SCHEDULE OF A CONCIERGE PHYSICIAN

Dr. Beth Willis opened a concierge practice two years ago. For ten years before that, she slaved away like Dr. Black. She finally got out of fast-food medicine and now structures her practice and time very differently. This is what her morning looks like:

9:00	Gene Davis	10:30	Wanda Samuelson
9:15		10:45	
9:30	Sharon Blair	11:00	Julie Powell
9:45		11:15	
10:00	Bill Williams	11:30	William Granite
10:15		11:45	

There are deliberate holes in Dr. Willis's schedule book. She typically sees only two or three patients every hour. She schedules only two patients per hour so that she can easily work someone in for an unexpected medical problem. If need be, she has 20 to 30 minutes to spend with a complex patient. Some hours, Dr. Willis schedules no patients at all in case she has to make a trip to the hospital or a house call.

Dr. Willis is available to her patients 24/7. She needs to be able to return pages or calls promptly. Because her patients pay her directly, she has a professional and a financial responsibility to be on call to protect them. She accepts no third-party payments for her services and sets her own rates. Medicare or HMOs do not control her fee structure nor, consequently, her schedule. In striving to protect her patients' health assets, her practice structure is more commensurate with her goals. Form follows function.

Dr. Willis still manages to see her own hospital patients, who love the continuity of care. She rounded on two of her hospital patients at 7:30 this morning and arrived in the office at 9 A.M. to see her first appointment. Her pace is much more leisurely than Dr. Black's. As she walks into her office, there are only two patients reading magazines in her waiting room, one for Dr. Willis and one for her partner. Dr. Willis's patient has not been waiting long. The staff promptly escorts the patient into Dr. Willis's examining room without making him spend another 15 minutes in "the second waiting room"—alone in a paper gown in a chilly exam room. The staff is professional and attentive. They appear to be happy in their work.

By lunchtime, Dr. Willis has seen only eight patients in her office instead of seventeen. One of her hospital patients developed an interesting and complex medical problem this morning, so she decides to order lunch in and read more about the problem. She logs on to a sophisticated computer program and reviews the most recent medical literature on the treatment of methicillin-resistant staph infections. She doesn't spend her time pandering to drug reps and get her drug information from a salesman anymore. This was one of the bad habits she abandoned when she opened her concierge practice.

During her lunch hour, Dr. Willis is very productive. She remembers how much fun mastering a complex medical problem can be. She has returned to that process of lifelong learning that was promised to her during medical school. She is delighted to find some new information. She calls the nurse at the hospital and alters the antibiotics for her patient. She feels good about her expanding professional knowledge.

After lunch, Dr. Willis returns to seeing patients in her office. One of her concierge patients calls with a sudden rash so she works him into an opening in the schedule. She then sees another patient who is suffering from depression and uses the extra time to listen. After the visit, she calls the mother of one of her pediatric patients to make sure the child's fever has come down. She returns some phone calls, speaking with an elderly patient who wants to know the results of her most recent CT scan.

Dr. Willis makes little more than Dr. Black, but she is much happier with the care she delivers to her patients. She likes her professional life. This spills over into her personal life. She spends more time with her family. As a result, she has a more balanced life.

Dr. Willis has more time to read and study medicine, so she feels like she is constantly becoming a better doctor. She has more knowledge to share with her patients. Less pressured, she is able to empathize with another human being who is in trouble.

THE SPACE BETWEEN LINES

If you were able to look between the lines on the scheduling sheets above, you would see that there is much more going on behind the scenes for both Dr. Black and Dr. Willis. They do much more than see patients during the day. They answer phone calls from other doctors, direct their staff, return pages, and dictate progress notes for each patient after every visit. This is why the typical office visit becomes far less than the 15 minutes allotted to the patient—the average person in this country spends only 8–12 minutes with his or her doctor. You can't create time where it does not exist.

In addition, both doctors will have to discuss difficult problems with specialists during the day. They will have to work in patients with immediate problems. Both doctors will have to make time to talk to worried family members about their sick loved ones. They will have to call in drugs to pharmacies. The list goes on and on.

If the time structure of a practice is already overburdened, these additional stresses will cause it to crack. Dr. Black now hates to be interrupted by the cardiologist who calls to talk about his patients. In his mind, there is no longer any such thing as "an interesting patient." As he listens to his cardiology colleague on the phone talk about one of his elderly patients, he feels tired and distracted. He is thinking, *Just do what you have to do. This is your specialty. I'll treat his diabetes.*

Furthermore, Dr. Black no longer has the luxury of thinking about his patients as complete human beings. Time pressure results in the farming out of their body parts to specialists. When a patient has chest pain, Dr. Black doesn't have time to go into a careful history but just refers most chest pain problems to the cardiologist, even if the chest pain may not be coming from the heart. He is not paid to be thorough. *Besides,* he thinks, *if it's the heart, let the specialist fight with the HMO about any needed procedures. If I order a thallium scan, the HMO will only deny it and require the cardiology consult anyway.* Tragically, Dr. Black has become a gatekeeper instead of a physician, reduced to a portal of entry to a complex system of approvals and denials.

TIME TO BE THOROUGH AND PROFESSIONAL

In contrast, when Dr. Willis gets a call from a cardiologist in the middle of her day, she has the time to talk. She is interested in what the cardiologist has to say—in fact, she's been reading about her patient's problem. This is a chance to collaborate and see the problem from another perspective. She is still the captain of her patient's medical team and so has scheduled safety valves into her day for this kind of professional exchange. Because she expects and plans for physician calls, these are not interruptions. A phone consultation with a colleague is an opportunity to learn and brainstorm. It improves patient care. It is one of the true joys of practicing medicine.

This contrast between Dr. Willis and Dr. Black may sound a bit contrived. Let me assure you that it is not. I know dozens of Dr. Blacks in Tucson, where I live. I once practiced like Dr. Black. As you will read in Chapter 7, I tried to change this broken system but was unsuccessful and so left this system for a better way. Now my life is much like that of Dr. Willis.

It is sad that many physicians like Dr. Black are just marking time until they can quit medicine or retire. What is equally sad is the limited care that patients receive as a result of these high-volume practices.

If you wouldn't invest your money in an unsound company, why would you entrust your most precious asset to a faulty medical system?

DOORKNOB SYNDROME

At this point, you get the picture that Dr. Black doesn't lead a very glamorous life. But you still may not be convinced that this could have a negative impact on you. You may think, "Who cares? We all work hard. Doctors still make a reasonable living, and there are plenty of worse jobs. So what if the doctor has to see so many patients?" Besides, maybe you're pretty healthy. How does this really affect you? Let's take a closer look at what might happen to you if something unexpected were to happen to your health.

There is a well-known phenomenon in medicine called "doorknob syndrome." Here's an example of how it works. Dr. Black is just about to end his 9 o'clock visit with a busy, forty-four-year-old CPA and mother of two, Sheryl Smith. Sheryl has been scheduled for a routine 15-minute office visit, ostensibly for a refill of her blood pressure medications and to have a blood pressure check. Everything looks fine. Dr. Black chats briefly with Mrs. Smith about her family. This will be an easy visit. As he puts his hand on the doorknob, Sheryl says, "Oh, by the way, Dr. Black, I think I may have a small lump in my breast. It's probably nothing. Maybe you don't even need to look at it today. It can wait until my next visit."

Sheryl is an extremely busy and successful businesswoman. She runs her own accounting firm of thirty-six employees. She's always been healthy and hasn't invested in finding a doctor who has time for his patients—she's too busy building a solid financial future for her family. So she gets her care through a low-cost insurer, the same one she uses for her employees. This keeps her overhead low.

She hasn't had a mammogram in two years. Dr. Black advised her to schedule one last year, but he didn't follow up with her or have his staff schedule one, and she has been "too busy at the office." The real reason

Sheryl doesn't get regular mammograms is fear. She is in denial. Her mother died of breast cancer at age forty-eight. Sheryl doesn't want to even entertain the possibility that this could happen to her.

Doorknob syndrome is common in all medical practices. Patients are often hesitant to bring up the real reason they made the appointment. Only at the end of the visit does the truth come out. Problems that are difficult for patients to face include breast lumps, depression, excessive drinking, or a sexually transmitted disease. When patients are scared, they need to talk. These problems are never easy. They cannot be handled quickly.

Presented with a case of doorknob syndrome involving possible breast cancer, Dr. Black finds himself pulled in two directions. He knows that Sheryl desperately needs his time—the one thing he doesn't have enough of. She needs a careful breast exam, a mammogram, and an ultrasound. Equally important, she needs some comfort and reassurance that Dr. Black will do whatever is necessary to help her. She wants to know what to expect. What tests will he order? What if she does have cancer? What will happen to her business and her family? Her mind begins to race.

What does Dr. Black do? There is no time for all of this. He begins to feel a knot tighten in his stomach. He knows he has a waiting room full of patients. He decides that he must be efficient with Sheryl. He prioritizes. He does a quick exam and identifies a suspicious mass. He tells Sheryl, "Don't worry just yet." He has his staff schedule a mammogram and an ultrasound, using the radiology company required by the discount insurance company. There will be a two-week wait for the mammogram. He schedules a follow-up appointment for Sheryl in three weeks. Depending on the mammogram, she may need a biopsy.

Dr. Black does what is absolutely necessary from a medical point of view. He delivers the "standard of care" for Sheryl within the limits of his practice structure. He will know what to do for Sheryl in three to four weeks. The time between visits will be torture for Sheryl and her worried family, but what else can he do?

During this encounter, there has been no time for emotional support. Dr. Black feels bad but rationalizes that it is partly her fault. After all, she should have mentioned it at the beginning of her visit, when at least there would have been a little more time.

Does Dr. Black want to limit care to Sheryl? Of course not! He feels uncomfortable with this. He is married. He wouldn't want his own wife treated this way. In fact, if this were to happen to his wife or mother, he'd call his oncology buddy who would see his wife immediately, give her lots of time, care, and support and expedite the diagnostics. However, Dr. Black has to live in the real world, under the restrictions of Sheryl's managed-care plan and its impact on his practice.

Dr. Black is now already 15 minutes behind schedule. His next patient is a seventy-five-year-old man with chronic congestive heart failure, diabetes, and coronary artery disease who is on eight different medications. He speaks little English and rarely goes to the lab for his required blood tests. He was just discharged from the hospital. There is no discharge summary from the hospitalist yet. Dr. Black has no idea what went on during the last hospital admission. The patient's new Medicare Part D drug plan requires prior authorization for one of his new, expensive heart medications. No time to talk with Sheryl any longer. Dr. Black has to forget about her problems and move on.

In Dr. Black's practice structure, the building is caving in. It is falling in on him and his patient, Sheryl. The elderly man with heart failure will see him only briefly.

A CONCIERGE APPROACH TO MRS. SMITH

If Sheryl were to present to Dr. Willis instead of Dr. Black, how might things be different? When a patient like Sheryl tells Dr. Willis about the breast lump, she takes her hand off the doorknob, sits down, and looks into her patient's eyes instead of avoiding them. Sheryl is clearly terrified; tears begin to well up as she speaks about her mother's death from breast cancer.

Dr. Willis has the time to deal with Sheryl as a person. She sets aside any discussions of mammograms or ultrasounds for the moment and simply *listens* to Sheryl. She shows empathy. Then she carefully examines her and feels the lump. A diagnosis must be made quickly.

Dr. Willis leaves the room and calls a radiology colleague to schedule an immediate diagnostic mammogram and possible biopsy for Sheryl. For such cases, Dr. Willis uses a group of radiologists who specialize in women's health and employ a new technology of rapid breast cancer diagnosis, a procedure embraced by medicine but not yet authorized by many HMOs. In some cases, a mammogram can be followed by a needle biopsy the same day, with results given to the patient within a matter of hours. This saves patients like Sheryl weeks of worry and heartache.

Three days later, the results are in. Sheryl's mammogram and biopsy are abnormal. She has been given a diagnosis of breast cancer. It is difficult news, but instead of waiting three agonizing weeks for it, Sheryl can immediately begin treatment. Dr. Willis sets up an appointment with Sheryl and her husband the next day, where they spend 45 minutes reviewing all of the treatment options of mastectomy vs. lumpectomy and radiation. Dr. Willis selects an excellent oncologist who she feels will also be a good personality match for Sheryl and makes a referral to a surgeon who specializes in breast surgery. Sheryl can talk to Dr. Willis, the oncologist, and the surgeon about her options. If she wishes, she can start attending a support group and discuss her concerns with other cancer survivors. She will get ongoing support from Dr. Willis.

As for doorknob syndrome, even if Sheryl never summoned up the nerve on her own to mention her lump, Dr. Willis always has the time to ask each patient a simple and powerful question: "Is there anything else you wanted to bring up today?"

HANDLING COMPLEX AND SENSITIVE MEDICAL PROBLEMS

Handling a problem like breast cancer is a sensitive issue. It is a problem that one in eight women will face in her lifetime. The treatment options must be discussed with the patient at their own pace. People process information differently, especially under these difficult circumstances. The best person to start those discussions is a qualified internist or family practitioner who really knows the patient. Of course, the oncologist's and surgeon's help is invaluable. Primary care doctors do not perform breast surgery or give radiation or chemotherapy. However, the opinions of a surgeon or an oncologist do not replace the role of the patient's personal physician.

I have personally diagnosed many women with breast cancer. The quality of mammography services in Tucson varies widely. I use true experts in this area, the best specialists available.

It takes time to go through this challenging period with a patient. If she needs a second opinion, it must be arranged. If she needs a third opinion in a difficult situation, the concierge physician should facilitate it.

Often, cancer treatment isn't black and white but can have many shades of gray. Some treatments, as for breast cancer, are based upon large, randomized controlled clinical trials and are relatively straight-forward. However, in other forms of cancer, treatment is more of an art. There may be little good information on the best therapy for less common tumors. One expert in oncology may approach the same cancer patient very differently than another would. The role of the concierge physician is to help the patient with the medical decision-making process. It is his job to get his hands on the very best numbers available, to listen to specialists with conflicting views and try to sort out any bias, and to explain to the patient what all of this information means and help them with their decisions.

PROSTATE CANCER

Though I have given you an example of breast cancer to illustrate the need for time with your doctor, prostate cancer in men is another example of a common and complex problem in which the role of the concierge physician is invaluable. Prostate cancer is a heterogeneous disease, meaning it is not a singular disease but a type of disease. It behaves differently at different ages. It can be aggressive in one man and slow growing in another. There are many strategies for treating prostate cancer, including no therapy at all. Men facing prostate cancer need the same time and resources as a woman facing breast cancer.

One of the greatest differences between concierge medicine and fast-food medicine is the personal responsibility the concierge doctor takes for managing the patient in totality. This is what all internists used to do. This is what I was trained to do at Cornell.

I was taught to value and use consultants for their special expertise. But I was also warned not to abdicate my medical responsibility by turning care over to the specialist. This principle has served me well over the years. I don't pretend to be smarter than a specialist in his or her area. I trust good specialists and select them very carefully. But I always verify by going back to the literature and asking questions. I frequently discuss treatment options with my specialists.

DEALING WITH THE INFORMATION EXPLOSION

Keeping up with new medical information is a critical issue for any conscientious doctor. This is of particular concern for the generalist, the internist, the family practitioner, or the pediatrician. According to the National Library of Medicine, between 1,500 and 3,500 completed medical references are added to the library every day. Literally thousands of new articles are added each week. To say that there is an information explosion is a gross understatement.

Clearly, doctors need to be more directed and efficient in their reading. They need to develop new skills in asking and answering pertinent clinical questions. However, they need time to do this. When they have more time to study a problem, they can investigate it at a deeper level. To stay up to speed, doctors need to structure reading time into their busy day. If doctors don't keep reading voraciously, their skills atrophy. This is no good for the patient; it is no good for the doctor. Schedules like Doctor Black's erode the knowledge base of the physician.

AFTER CANCER THERAPY

After a cancer diagnosis, a concierge doctor continues to be involved in his patient's total care. For example, Dr. Willis might notice that a patient like Sheryl is a little overweight. From her history, we know that she has become very sedentary since opening her own firm. Dr. Willis would explain the most recent literature on body weight, diet, and exercise in breast cancer recovery. She would discuss the role of exercise in recovering breast cancer patients and dispel old myths about avoiding strength training in cancer patients.

Dr. Willis might offer Sheryl assistance with a nutrition and exercise program to lose 10 pounds of excess body fat. Sheryl would begin to feel more in control of her own life. She would no longer be the passive object of an impersonal cancer treatment machine, a person who is having things done to her. Instead, she would be taking an active role in her care, investing in her health in more ways than one.

Sheryl might ask Dr. Willis about some alternative medicine remedies that she has read about for breast cancer on the Internet. Dr. Willis might take the information, review it, and make a follow-up appointment in which she'd explain to Sheryl that there is little science behind these particular approaches but also encourage her to explore any and all avenues that interest her as long as she didn't rely on untested therapies for something as serious as cancer.

Alice in Wonderland

If reading these contrasting stories about Sheryl sounds like Alice through the looking glass, let me assure you that they are based in fact. The story of Sheryl Smith is taken from my own patients, both before and after I started practicing concierge medicine seven years ago. When I practiced like Dr. Black, I had little time to do more than refer my patients to an oncologist or surgeon for their cancer care. When they had questions, I referred them back to their oncologists. In treating patients under a concierge model, I have been more involved. I have been in situations in which many specialists had conflicting opinions and I acted as the referee. I have found third or even fourth opinions.

I have also become an expert in writing exercise prescriptions for cancer patients. I am often referred cancer patients by private oncologists so that they may exercise under my supervision in an exercise studio in my office. Oncologists at the Arizona Cancer Center have recently come to me for advice on how to individualize cancer survivorship programs. We are working on plans to teach their residents and fellows how to integrate exercise physiology into the care of their cancer patients.

HOW MY TIME IS USED

Concierge medicine provides me with the structure to help my patients truly invest in their health. It provides the following benefits:

- More time for the doctor and the patient during visits.
- More time for the doctor to study and read.
- More time for the doctor to consult with specialists.
- More time to think about complex medical problems.
- Time for the doctor to act as teacher.
- Time for the doctor to go beyond crisis care and talk about wellness, especially after a diagnosis of cancer or other serious health threats.
- More time to individualize a recovery plan.
- More time to absorb those inevitable disasters that affect every doctor's day.

- Finally, more time for the doctor to care for himself; the last thing you want is a doctor who is not in charge of his own health assets and functions suboptimally.

The Executive Physical

In addition to longer office visits, most concierge doctors also offer some form of an "executive physical." I spend about 2 hours with my new patients during their initial visit. By contrast, most initial comprehensive visits with a conventional doctor are scheduled for only 30 to 45 minutes, depending on the age of the patient.

A young doctor I once hired as an associate asked me, "What do you do with a new patient for 2 hours?" Good question.

- I sit down and review all of their old records. I do this with the patient in front of me so I can ask questions to clarify the medical history.
- I take my own careful history from the patient, letting them talk and tell me about their problems in their own words. I am not just being cordial. It is good medicine. This process often leads to the consideration of other diagnoses.
- I take an in-depth family history and a thorough social history. I want to know who this patient is and what makes them tick.
- I take an exercise and nutrition history.
- I carefully examine the patient. It is not a superficial 5-minute affair.
- A comprehensive blood panel is drawn in my office.
- I perform a stress test on my patients. I do the test myself so that I can observe the patient under the stress of exercise rather than turn this over to a technician who does not understand exercise physiology. Neither do I send them to a cardiologist's office where a medical assistant will run the stress test.
- I perform a body composition test.
- I consider any special tests that may be appropriate given the patient's history and exam. I answer a patient's questions about such things as CT scans of the heart and total body CT scans.
- All healthcare maintenance is addressed during the visit, including studies like a mammogram or colonoscopy.
- Vaccinations are brought up to date.
- After all of this information is put together, I sit down with the patient and give them a summary of my initial impressions. We set goals. We

schedule a formal exercise and fitness consultation. We schedule a follow-up visit. We create an investment plan to increase the value of their health assets.

This is what takes 2 hours in my executive physical. Contrast this to a 30-minute routine office physical: 15 minutes for the history, 15 minutes for the exam, and you're done.

CONCIERGE MEDICINE FOR THE FAMILY

I am not a family practitioner. I care for some older children of sixteen to eighteen years at the request of their parents, but I do not see many children. A family practitioner or pediatrician who opts for a concierge style of practice would use the same principles of time and access in caring for children.

Is there a need for concierge care for kids? Do I think that investing in a child's health is a good idea? Absolutely! Just look at the number of obese children who are walking around your local shopping mall. Pay attention to those articles in the newspaper about the dramatic rise in type 2 diabetes among teenagers. This epidemic of obesity, sedentary lifestyle, and poor nutrition is having a profoundly detrimental impact on the precious asset of our children's health. And what about substance abuse and the complex issue of teenage sexuality? How can you deal with these problems in a brief visit, along with all of the routine and not-so-routine care? Kids need time as well.

If you want concierge care for your children, look around. If you have a child who is battling a difficult problem like obesity, find someone with the time to design a tailored exercise and nutritional plan to meet their needs. If your child has severe asthma and her care is fragmented and disorganized, look for a doctor who will take you out of the third-party practice model. Get some individual attention.

As I've said throughout this book, concierge medicine is a patient-driven process. It is relatively new. If there are no pediatricians or family practitioners offering this service in your area now, talk to your doctor. Be creative. These programs will come.

I used to run a childhood obesity program in a fitness facility next door to my office. The stories were tragic. I have seen several obese teenagers at the request of their overworked pediatricians. I've seen twelve-year-old girls who weighed 240 pounds. I've spoken with the parents of these children and realized that you cannot treat the child without involving the entire family. You just can't deal effectively with a complex problem like childhood obesity in a routine pediatric office visit. If left untreated, the problem will only get worse and create a lifetime of liabilities for the child.

THE CONCIERGE PHYSICIAN AS GENERALIST

People often don't understand the true value of a generalist in medicine. They think they can get great medical care in modern medicine by using a bunch of specialists. I disagree. A well-trained internist does not have the depth of knowledge in oncology that the oncologist has or the cardiac knowledge of the cardiologist, but this does not mean that all cardiac care should be turned over to the cardiologist. When I was at UCLA, the chief of cardiology said that he believed 85 percent of cardiology care should be returned to the internist. I agree.

The internist is expert at looking at the whole patient and seeing the connection among the parts. He has a wide breadth and depth of knowledge in all of the subspecialties of internal medicine. He can evaluate clinical trials, just like a specialist can. He can use most cardiac medications, just like the cardiologist. He treats thyroid problems, diabetes, infections, heart disease, and many other problems.

The generalist has a good working knowledge of all of the subspecialties of medicine and knows how to integrate the care of multiple body systems. When a heart patient goes on chemotherapy that might adversely affect the heart, the internist is in a unique position to carefully follow the patient and make recommendations.

It is also important to remember that subspecialists in our current healthcare system are very busy. Many of them are playing the volume game in their offices, seeing as many patients as they possibly can. An internist or generalist with the time can search the literature on a complex problem, consult with world-class specialists, and often come up with an answer that an overworked specialist may not have the time to research. This happens frequently in my practice.

I don't pretend to be smarter than the specialist or to have the same working knowledge in his area of expertise, but I am board-certified in internal medicine, and oncology and cardiology are subspecialties in my area. When I find a new drug or treatment option that my specialists have not considered, I call them and ask questions. My specialists thank me when I do this kind of legwork for them. We work together as a team. We don't play hot potato with the patient, tossing him back and forth from doctor to doctor.

Probably the single greatest difference between a generalist in an HMO model and a generalist who practices concierge medicine is a return to the status of the medical quarterback. As opposed to being a referral source for specialists, a concierge doctor is the person who calls the medical plays. He orchestrates all of the action on the field.

AMA ETHICAL GUIDELINES ON CONCIERGE MEDICINE

The AMA has taken the position that there is nothing intrinsically unethical about concierge medicine. However, they are careful to point out that doctors should not advertise this form of medicine as a means to provide "better diagnostic or therapeutic care." I understand what the AMA is saying here. In general, I agree with them. We should not give the impression that the only way to get good care is for the patient to pay a concierge or retainer fee or that concierge doctors are "better physicians." Plenty of people get excellent care in our traditional system, despite its flaws. Others do not.

However, I must be honest with you. I must be honest with myself. I believe that a model like Dr. Willis's offers better patient care than Dr. Black's. Since I have changed the structure of my practice, I have had more time to study medicine. I am more up-to-date than I was when I was seeing thirty patients a day. I also have more flexibility to adapt to new medical discoveries than I did then.

As an example, I recently saw a patient who had a recurrence of a small lung tumor. She was not a candidate for lung surgery and did not want chemotherapy. With some research, I found a local specialist performing a new technique called radio frequency ablation, in which a small wire is placed in a tumor without the need for open chest surgery. High-frequency radio waves then "cook" the tumor and kill it. It works well for many small lung tumors. Few Tucson doctors even know about the local availability of this cutting-edge technique. However, having more time to look under all the rocks and find new and creative solutions to problems, I became aware of this treatment option, could read the literature before suggesting it to my patient, and called an expert at Brown University to discuss his vast experience in radio frequency ablation. It made a big difference for my patient. I just couldn't do this if, like Dr. Black, I were still seeing thirty patients per day.

In general, most patients eventually get the same diagnostic and therapeutic decisions in either medical model. However, there are clearly exceptions in which doctors who have more time are able to deliver better care. In general, I believe that more time allows professionals to do a better job. If I didn't believe this were true, I wouldn't practice concierge medicine.

We need to respect the spirit of the AMA guidelines, especially in mixed concierge practices like mine. We do not want to deliver different levels of care based upon payment. In my practice, my schedule allows me to give more time to all of my patients—including indigent patients. We must be honest about the importance of time in providing good care.

THE CRITICAL FACTOR OF TIME

Whether you are dealing with breast cancer, a heart problem, an infection, or any other serious illness, you are confronting a medical crisis. You are dealing with a very real threat to your most precious asset. Understand that your doctor's practice and the way that he structures his time will have a direct impact on his ability to protect you.

When you develop a serious medical problem, you are not just dealing with an insult to your tissue. Serious medical problems often cause great fear. Fear attacks your spirit. It attacks your ability to think clearly. You need a doctor with the time and expertise to help you manage that fear and think clearly about your options.

If your doctor does not have the time to support you, you will be left to your own resources. If medical decisions are made in haste, if you fail to get the very best advice available, if you fail to turn over the right stone, you may pay a big price.

In the broad scheme of things, concierge medicine is a small investment, especially given the potential return on that investment.

CHAPTER 6

Your Exercise Portfolio

FINANCIAL INVESTING

When people have money left over from the expenses of daily living, such as the cost of their housing, food, and other necessities, they have what is called *capital*. The sole purpose of investing is to make that capital grow. The result of the successful growth of capital is what most people call wealth.

People typically invest their capital in a number of different investment vehicles. They don't put all of their eggs in one basket. These vehicles may include stocks, bonds, real estate, and other investments. Many people are fearful about investing in individual stocks, so they invest in mutual funds. A mutual fund is a group of stocks or securities that is managed by what the investor hopes is an *expert*.

The sum of your financial investments is what is called your financial portfolio. When the value of one of your investments falls, the value of your portfolio drops. Depending upon how much money you have in a failing investment, the value of your portfolio will drop proportionately.

Your *health portfolio* is very much like your financial portfolio. It is made up of multiple assets. Your body's overall health is dependent upon the optimal functioning of each of its assets, which we call bodily systems. Depending on the combined strength of these systems, your body is either in good health or in poor health. These systems include:

- Your cardiovascular system (your heart and blood vessels)
- Your nervous system (your brain, spinal cord and nerves, and its by-products, which you call your "mind" and your "psychological health")
- Your reproductive system (including your sexual and reproductive organs)
- Your musculoskeletal system (your muscles and bones)
- Your endocrine system (your pituitary gland, thyroid gland, adrenal glands, testicles, ovaries, and other organs that secrete vital hormones)
- Your hematopoietic system (your white and red blood cells, along with platelets)
- Your pulmonary system (your lungs and airways that supply oxygen to all your body's cells)

Remember, I define "wellness" in practical terms. *Wellness is a human performance issue.* Why should this definition have any value to you? I use this definition of wellness because it is practical. It is functional. You can use it to measure and follow your sense of wellness objectively.

By improving just two vital parameters of your body's performance, your *strength* and your *endurance*, you indirectly increase the value of *all* of your health assets in the process. When you are stronger and have a sense of reserve, you feel well. If you become fitter, not only will your muscles, bones, and heart work better; every system in your body will work better including your brain, which is the very essence of who you are. All of your health assets will increase in value.

TWO COMMON MYTHS SURROUNDING EXERCISE

Before I go any further, I would like to dispel two common myths that people have about exercise, or the lack thereof:

- "The only reason to exercise is to get fitter. I don't need to be fitter. I am happy just staying the same."
- "Any amount of exercise that I do will significantly improve my health."

First, it is worth repeating the fact that at any point in time, we are either in the process of getting stronger or getting weaker. It is very difficult to stay the same. If you are not in the process of getting stronger, your strength and endurance are slowly deteriorating over time. In addition, so are the bodily systems that support your strength.

Second, though any amount of exercise is better than living a completely sedentary life, many people delude themselves into thinking that they are improving their health significantly by simply walking to work, doing a little gardening, or taking a leisurely stroll.

MEASURING FINANCIAL PERFORMANCE OVER TIME

If you examine the financial performance of a group of stocks over time, like the NASDAQ index, you will frequently see the numbers displayed in a curve. Even if you don't like curves, stay with me. They are easy to understand. Curves are used to evaluate performance because they allow us to look at trends. They answer a critical question: Are the numbers looking better or are they looking worse over a period of time? Is the performance of my investments trending upward or is it trending downward? Am I getting an increasing return on my investments or am I losing money?

If your stock performance is weakening over time, you will want to change your investment strategy. If your portfolio shows a downward slope, your assets are depreciating. As any financial investor will tell you, growth is everything. If your money is not growing, you are wasting your capital.

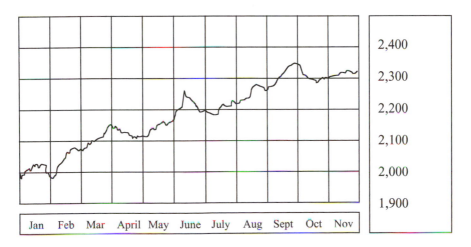

TRACKING PERSONAL HEALTH

Similarly, your health is a form of capital that you'll want to grow over time. When you make regular investments of exercise, your primary purpose is to grow your health. *You are simply using exercise as an investment vehicle to reach your goal of greater health.*

At the end of a three-month investment period, you should be stronger than you were when you started. You will want to be healthier. This is why I advise people to exercise. Don't exercise for exercise's sake—that is, unless you really like it! Exercise to get stronger. Exercise to grow your health assets and get real results. To this end, make sure that you have a reasonable plan.

As a doctor, I can draw curves that track the performance of your health portfolio. I can trace a simple curve of your strength over time. This is just what a financial advisor does with your money. Tracking your progress, whether it is with money or fitness, is how you can tell if your investment strategy is working.

When you exercise, think of each session as making a small deposit into your health portfolio. If done properly, you should get a return on each investment of time and effort.

Here is what a health portfolio assessment looks like for a successful health investor.

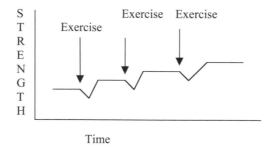

Notice that after each deposit of exercise, there is a little dip downward. There is a temporary decrease in strength after an exercise investment. You experience a little fatigue after exercise. This is normal. As I will explain later, this is a necessary part of growth. After the small dip, there is an improvement in strength, which takes you to a new level. This improvement in strength occurs during a period of rest.

Over time, the successful health investor is becoming physically stronger. His rate of growth is slow and steady. At the end of a three-month period, he is much stronger than when he started investing. Though this curve shows only the single parameter of strength over time, *all* of the investor's health assets are appreciating in value as she gets stronger. Why do I say this? How can all of your health assets increase in value just because you are getting stronger?

You cannot develop stronger muscles and bones without creating a stronger heart to supply blood to these muscles. You cannot become stronger without producing more red blood cells to carry more oxygen to your muscles. To get stronger, you will also need more tiny blood vessels, called capillaries, to carry those red blood cells to your working muscles. The lining of your blood vessels, called the endothelium, will improve in function, decreasing your risk of heart attack and stroke. As you become fitter and as all of these changes take place, your body is able to operate more efficiently. Your resting heart rate drops. You feel more at ease. You sleep better. Your resistance to disease is increased. You slow the process of physiologic aging. Your endocrine system is in better balance. Glucose is metabolized more efficiently. You feel better emotionally. Your brain works better. Your libido and sex drive increase. Your posture improves. You look better! All of your bodily systems improve as your strength improves. Strength is just a *marker* of your appreciating assets.

RATE OF GROWTH

If your health is poor to begin with, don't worry. This just means that your initial gains will be proportionately much greater than those of a highly fit person who is working toward marginal gains in performance. As long as you keep investing, your health will continue to grow. It is no different than growing your money.

In a fascinating study of debilitated ninety-year-old nursing home patients, tremendous gains in strength were reported with just twelve weeks of a strength training investment. In this landmark study published in the *New England Journal of Medicine*, frail elderly patients increased their leg strength by over 100 percent in just three months of weight training. This study demonstrates the principle that those who are the weakest have the most to gain by exercising. In contrast, an Olympic athlete, who is highly fit, works very hard for tiny gains in strength and performance. This is why I tell unfit people not to be discouraged. They have a lot to look forward to. Building strength is different than building wealth in this regard. In wealth, the rich get richer much faster than the poor because they have more capital to start with. The opposite is true with fitness.

A 100 percent gain in strength is a pretty nice rate of return on a three-month investment. For these sedentary nursing home residents, an increase in strength resulted in greater personal freedom. They could walk more easily. Their gait strength and walking speed improved. They functioned more independently. They felt better. Their improved strength resulted in greater independence to move about in their world. It reduced the risks of falls, hip fractures, and other disabilities. This study also demonstrates that you are never too old to start investing in your health.

STAGNATING HEALTH CAPITAL

Here is a strength curve for people who do not invest in their most precious asset.

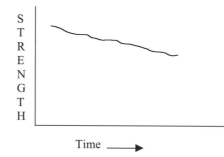

The strength of these people is slowly declining over time. At the same time that they are getting weaker, their other bodily systems are also depreciating. They may be developing atherosclerotic plaques in their blood vessels. These plaques are deposited in their brain, their heart, and other critical blood vessels. They may develop premature heart disease as a result. They may suffer an early stroke. As they get weaker and feel less vital, they may experience a loss of libido. Their sexual performance diminishes. As they look in the mirror, they feel bad about what they see. They may begin to experience mild symptoms of depression. With the passage of time, the value of all of their health assets plummets.

This depreciating investment curve is what I call the "default curve." By default, I mean that with no action taken, there are predictable negative consequences. There is a slow and steady devaluation of health assets. This "noninvestor" allows gravity and age to take their toll. The individual is not getting better over time. She is getting worse. No matter what vitamins or supplements she takes, she cannot *feel* better. Health performance does not come in a bottle. It comes from investing in yourself!

THE PASSIVE INVESTOR

The third investment curve is of someone who goes through the motions of investing in exercise, but does so without a good plan or a goal.

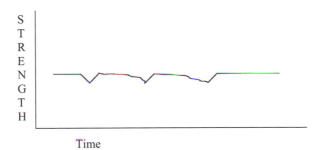

This is the curve of the *passive, intermittent* investor. This is the person who exercises sporadically at low levels, without a well-crafted plan. This person exercises without a specific goal in mind. This person does not understand the basic concepts of exercise investing. Such people do not put in enough effort to get an improvement in their strength.

This same result occurs when a well-intentioned person hires a bad "personal trainer." Many people work out with bad trainers and get little out of their investment of time and money. The personal trainer behaves like a mediocre financial consultant. The trainer's knowledge base is limited. They charge a usual and customary fee for training, but they do not help the client to invest with a purpose. If you are involved with such a trainer, your health will not grow. You are wasting precious health capital, not to mention time and money, with such an advisor. You should find a good trainer. There are plenty of good trainers out there. If possible, look for someone who has formal training in exercise science.

Good trainers are invaluable in health investing. A good trainer can be used to work in cooperation with a concierge physician.

THE SIMPLE SECRET OF SUCCESSFUL EXERCISE INVESTING

Now that you've seen a couple of different strength curves, I am going to explain the single most important concept in health investing. If you grasp its importance, you will be far ahead of the game. If you can *apply* the concept to each of your workouts, you will experience steady gains in your progress. This concept is what exercise specialists call the *overload principle*.

What the overload principle says is that to get stronger, you have to ask your body to do something that it cannot easily do. When you put a stress on your body in the form of exercise, your body must rise to the occasion. It tries to meet the extra load that you place on it. It works harder until it fails. When you then give your body rest after overloading it, it becomes stronger! Simple, right? Let's look at the first curve that I drew, in more detail, to better understand the overload principle.

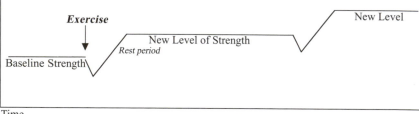

Notice that immediately after exercise, the body is a little weaker than when it started. If you've ever worked out, you know exactly what I mean. If you do a workout at your local gym, you will feel a little weaker at the end of your session than you did at the beginning. If you tried to repeat the same workout twice in the same day without rest, you couldn't get through the full workout the second time around. You would be spent.

During the critical period of rest, the body mobilizes all of its resources to become stronger. During this period, you are building new muscle tissue. You are forming new blood vessels to meet the increased demands. Your nervous system is learning to fire coordinated electrical impulses more effectively. Your heart is learning to function better as a pump. Your blood vessels learn to work more efficiently and in concert with your heart.

Resting, like sleep, is not merely a passive process. While you rest, your body is mobilizing all of its forces to get stronger. It is building new tissue, so that the next time you exercise, your body will be prepared to handle a greater stress. *While resting, you should be investing in your health by giving your body the nutrients that it needs to become stronger.* You need to make a nutritional investment to build healthy muscle and repair any minor damage that was done. This is why good nutrition is such a critical investment in your health. We will address the subject of nutrition in the next chapter.

Understanding the importance of good nutrition explains why fad diets, like the Atkins diet, are such a bad idea. A high-fat diet is poor in vital nutrients. It simply doesn't provide the building blocks that your assets need to grow. In fact, the late Dr. Robert Atkins understood that this was a problem with his diet. This is why he sold dozens of supplements on his Web site which he called "vita-nutrients." Even so, there is no evidence that such a strategy works.

AN UPWARD TREND

After a period of rest and refueling, your next workout session becomes easier. You feel stronger because you *are* stronger. You *know* this is true because you can repeat the same exercise more times than you could during your previous workout. You may even be able to lift a heavier weight than you could in your previous training session. When done right, the improvements are slow and steady.

There is no quick investment strategy in the game of building health. It takes time; time to exercise and time to rest. Regardless of income, everybody plays by the same rules. These are nature's rules. Health investing is the great equalizer. There are no hedge funds, flipping of real estate, or other fast-track, high-risk investing options with your health.

This principle of overload may seem very simple to you. You may have even heard of this concept before. It is *simple*, but not always *easy* to implement. I know world-class athletes who don't put this principle to use effectively. They either exercise with an inadequate workload to grow or work out too hard, overtrain, and lose strength over time. They may not get the proper rest they need to recover before their next bout.

Similarly, many coaches and trainers believe in pushing people to their absolute limits, as if they were following some Hollywood boot camp script. This is nonsense. This approach just discourages people as they experience excessive soreness, chronic fatigue, and sometimes even injuries. Total exhaustion is not the goal! Slow improvement in strength and endurance is the goal.

HOW MUCH SHOULD YOU EXERCISE?

The answer to this question should be individualized and is contained within our simple overload graph. How fit do you want to become? How much do you want to invest? If you want to get *very* strong, you are going to have to make large investments of time and energy. You will need to get proper rest in between investments. You may be exhausted in between your exercise sessions, because you work very hard. The valley in your strength curve will be quite deep in this case. You will need adequate time to recover. This is what professional athletes do. They push the performance envelope. Most people do not have the time, money, or interest in having the performance assets of an Olympian. It is certainly not necessary for excellent health.

When you grasp the concept of the overload curve, you realize why I say *exercise must be tailored to meet the needs of the individual*. What may be an appropriate stress load for me may not be a proper exercise stress load for you, and vice versa. If you don't work out hard enough to stress your body, your assets will not grow. If you work out too hard, your body will break down over time. If you have a bad knee, the stress of running is not appropriate for your body. If you have diabetes, you will need to consider the impact of hypoglycemia, or low blood sugar, during your workouts. The individual considerations in determining how much you exercise are infinite.

However, if you get some expert advice from a professional who knows you and understands your personal goals, he or she can design an appropriate program for you. As a concierge physician, this is what I do. I also track the gains in strength and performance in my patients. I ask them to keep track of their progress during workouts. My patients keep exercise logs. If they have a personal trainer, I ask the trainer to periodically prepare a simple report for me. I look at their numbers over time. I look at their strength gains, or lack thereof. I make suggestions for new strategies that will increase health and vitality further.

If you just want to be moderately fit, which is where the greatest health return on investment is found, you don't need to kill yourself. You don't need to spend all of your time and effort exercising. After all, there are lots of other things that we need and want to do with our lives. Most of us want to spend time with our friends, spouses, and children. We want to do those things that bring us joy. We want some balance in our lives.

Most people are very busy. They need to be efficient. They need to exercise with the intent of getting the greatest returns on their investment of time. This is the reason to have a tailor-made program crafted by your health advisor.

ENDURANCE TRAINING: INTENSITY AND DURATION

The second part of your exercise investment strategy should focus on improving your endurance. The value of endurance has been recognized since ancient times. It has been said that the race goes not to the swiftest, nor the strongest, but to the one who can endure. So true!

Endurance training involves a different kind of investment strategy than strength training. Endurance or aerobic exercises involve rhythmic, repetitive muscle contractions. Examples include brisk walking, jogging, cycling, swimming, or using aerobic equipment like an elliptical trainer. Endurance training is critical for good cardiovascular health.

We use different parameters to determine whether or not an investment of endurance exercise is paying off. Endurance training does not allow you to lift heavier weights. It allows you to go longer. As I noted previously, the time you last on a standard treadmill test is an excellent way to track the progress of your endurance investment.

Objective assessments of endurance are more reliable than taking an exercise history. Many people come to my office and tell me how much aerobic exercise they do. They may say, "I run 3 miles every day" or "I walk for half an hour three times per week." However, these statements give me little objective information about their endurance. This information doesn't tell me what I need to know to help a person with their investment. If you say that you run 3 miles, do you run three 7-minute miles or do you jog/walk three 15-minute miles? When you walk for 30 minutes, do you stroll with your arthritic, fourteen-year-old Cocker Spaniel, or do you power walk with your teenage grandson?

There are two important parameters in all forms of aerobic exercise: the *intensity* of your aerobic exercise and the *duration* of the exercise session. Your body does not know how many miles you walk or jog. It does not have a built-in odometer. Your body doesn't care about distance. All your body knows is *how hard* it is working and *how long* you are making it work that hard.

AEROBIC EXERCISE INTENSITY

There are two ways that you can measure your exercise intensity during aerobic exercise: you can estimate intensity by using "perceived exertion," or you can use a heart rate monitor.

To use the perceived exertion method, simply ask yourself how hard you feel like you are working on a scale of 1–10. If 1 is the easiest and 10 is the hardest you've ever worked out, you will want to do most aerobic workouts at an intensity of about 7/10. Now, if you were to tell me that you work out at a perceived exertion of 5/10 for 30 minutes, I can more appropriately advise you on what you might do to improve your aerobic exercise program to have more endurance.

If perceived exertion does not get the results you want, or if you would like to be more precise and scientific with your aerobic exercise, you can purchase an inexpensive heart rate monitor. Heart rate monitors serve the function of a tachometer on a car. All sports cars come with a tachometer. The tachometer does not tell the driver the speed at which he is moving. The tachometer tells the driver how hard his engine is working. There is a "redline" indicator on a tachometer above which the RPMs are so high that the engine is in danger of overheating. The same principle applies to using a heart rate monitor.

When you use a heart rate monitor, you can determine precisely how hard your heart is working at any moment in time. You can exercise at an appropriate intensity to stay within your prescribed "target zones." When your target heart rates are accurately set by your physician or other health professional, you become more efficient with your time. You get more out of each aerobic session. You also know when you are above your redline pulse. The heart rate monitor is like an exquisite biofeedback tool. It helps you to become more in tune with your body.

A WORD ABOUT TRAINING ZONES

There are many simple formulas available on the Internet and in exercise books to help you calculate how fast your heart rate should be during aerobic exercise. These formulas are based upon average heart rates in the population. These population norms are called nomograms. For example, the old saw that your maximum heart rate is 220 minus your age is just an approximation. This method will be incorrect for 33 percent of the population. This is why I measure my patients' maximum heart rate during a stress test. I don't want to be giving bad exercise advice to one-third of my patients. Their time is too precious to waste exercising at the wrong intensity.

Furthermore, if you take the estimated maximum heart rate and then arbitrarily exercise at 70 percent of this number, you may be exercising at the wrong intensity altogether. If you wish to get more precise, you will have to work with your concierge physician or other expert to determine your true training heart rates.

There is also a great deal of value in mixing up your aerobic exercise sessions. You shouldn't exercise at the same heart rate all the time. Optimally, one workout per week will be done for a longer duration at a lower intensity, to teach your body to burn fat as fuel more efficiently. In addition, I often prescribe one *interval training* session per week for patients wishing to improve their endurance. Interval training involves brief periods (30 seconds to 5 minutes) of high-intensity aerobics followed by several minutes of low-level, recovery activity. It is beyond the scope of this chapter to describe the technicalities of interval training. However, you should ask your physician about the efficiency of using this method to increase your return on investment. This useful investment tool is often left out of general exercise programs.

EXERCISE CLEARANCE

If you are a man over forty or a woman over fifty, you should also make sure that you have a physical examination and a stress test before you start a vigorous exercise program. If you have health problems, this assessment should be done at an earlier age. Consult your doctor!

From a statistical point of view, exercise is extraordinarily safe. However, to invest safely, you will want to get the help of a qualified doctor. Once you have the clearance to start your program, sit down with your doctor to develop an effective, efficient plan to maximize your results.

HOW OFTEN SHOULD YOU DO STRENGTH TRAINING AND ENDURANCE TRAINING?

There is no simple answer to this question. Instead, I will give you some general rules of thumb. First, you need to decide how much time you have to invest every week. Then you need to go back and look at those personal goals. If I am counseling a thirty-five-year-old woman who wants to lose 30 pounds and has only 3 hours per week to exercise, I am going to write an exercise prescription which focuses on endurance training. Why? Because minute for minute, aerobic exercise burns about twice as many calories as weight training burns. If the goal is weight loss, I will focus on burning calories first. I will advise getting stronger later.

On the other hand, if I have a seventy-year-old man who has been sedentary for years, I am going to focus his time and effort on rebuilding lost muscle mass and strength. His program will be weighted toward strength training. Aerobic training can come later.

The key in designing your personal exercise program is to find an expert advisor who knows how to tailor a plan to meet your needs. Generalized guidelines, like those put forth by major health organizations, have little value when applied to the individual. I've yet to meet the person who should follow the American College of Sports Medicine guidelines for general fitness literally. Apparently, the public agrees with me. Telling Americans for two decades that they should do three to five aerobic exercise sessions per week (20–60 minutes in their target zones) plus two weight training sessions per week plus stretching has accomplished little in the promotion of health. After twenty years of this message, less than 20 percent of the population follows the guidelines. General advice like this makes no more sense than telling the "average financial investor" that he or she should put 50 percent of his or her money in stocks, 25 percent in bonds, and 25 percent in gold. There is no such thing as the average investor, whether you are talking about growing health or wealth.

WHY IS EXERCISE SUCH A GREAT INVESTMENT?

Again, when you exercise effectively, you are not just building your strength and your endurance. You are measurably increasing the assets of all of your bodily systems. By getting stronger, you enhance the value of each individual asset in your health portfolio:

- You increase the amount of lean muscle in your asset column.
- You increase the number of energy-producing powerhouses in your cells— little organelles called mitochondria—which produce ATP.
- Your cardiovascular system is tuned up. You reach your "redline pulse" at a higher level of exertion than you did previously. You are more efficient when you idle.
- You increase your good cholesterol and lower your bad cholesterol.
- You improve the strength of your bones.
- You improve the way that your brain works.
- You sleep better.
- Your libido and sexual function improve.
- You metabolize glucose better, reducing your risk of diabetes.
- Your immune function improves.
- You reduce your physiologic age. You feel and look younger.

This is only a partial list of the valuable returns on investment that you get from simply getting stronger. All you need to do to get all of these benefits is to follow the simple overload theory. It is all in the curve.

If investing in your body is new to you, start out slowly. If you have been sedentary, start with a simple walking program. If you are already pretty fit, consider getting even stronger.

THE ROLE OF THE CONCIERGE DOCTOR

What I have done in this chapter is to provide you with some important concepts and general exercise guidelines. However, only your doctor can find the best way to apply these principles to your individual situation. Your concierge physician is the perfect person to help you with an initial health assessment. He is the appropriate person to provide clearance for an exercise program. Ideally, he will also be the person who helps you write your exercise program. He should follow your progress. He may suggest putting together a health investment team, using ancillary professionals like a qualified personal trainer or exercise physiologist and a registered dietician.

If you choose a concierge physician who does not have the expertise or willingness to help you with an exercise plan, you will have to supplement your health investment with additional professionals. Try looking for a qualified exercise physiologist in your community—preferably someone with a bachelor's, master's, or even a Ph.D. in exercise physiology. If your concierge physician does not do stress testing himself, have him refer you to a cardiologist.

Not everyone can easily find a concierge doctor who is expert in the details of crafting an exercise program. However, if you as the consumer request this service, your concierge doctor will ultimately respond to your needs. Doctors lacking in exercise and nutritional knowledge will ultimately have to take continuing medical education courses to bone up on these important topics. If they don't, they will lose patients. *All* people need this critical information for optimal health!

There is a lot of room for legitimate differences in the way that good medicine is practiced. I may use one antibiotic for a given infection, while a colleague may have an equally valid and different choice of drugs. However, the health benefits of some kind of regular activity are incontrovertible. If your doctor doesn't get this, you may have a problem.

This is *your* health. It is *your* asset. To make your asset grow, you will need to assemble the appropriate experts. If you default to the position of leading a sedentary lifestyle, if you fail to invest wisely, your health assets will surely depreciate. This is not a moralistic or judgmental statement; it is a law of nature. It is a statement that you can validate for yourself. Just look at the people around you. Most people who lead fit and active lives get more out of life, and it shows. Most overweight and sedentary people give off a different vibe. Get your inspiration from those who are strong, and follow their lead.

If you make health a priority, you can achieve great health. Exercise need not be intimidating. It need not be complex. Make small investments every week. Just remember the curve. You can do this with the help of your concierge doctor.

CHAPTER 7

A Lifelong Nutritional Strategy

BRICKS AND MORTAR

Imagine that you have the wealth to build your dream home. You find the right architect. You find a great builder. You buy a piece of property on a hill. You have the money set aside for the project. Months into construction, you are called by the builder. He tells you that there is a shortage of the flagstone that you chose for the face of your home. The builder suggests that you compromise. He asks you to substitute with products that are readily available. You reluctantly give up your plan for the entryway of your beautiful new home. You are disappointed. You have the dream; you even have the money. But you just don't have the raw materials that you need for construction.

Building your body is no different than building a home. Food provides the necessary building blocks for the body that you want. If you don't have the right raw materials, you can't create what you envision. Like other material possessions, houses come and go. However, your body is the only *home* that you will live in for the rest of your life. It deserves a good nutritional investment. You want your body to last. You want it to be comfortable to live in—warm in the winter, cool in the summer—and to look good. You don't want it to be plagued by things constantly going wrong that require time and money to fix, things that weaken the overall structure, sap your enjoyment, and make you worry about what is going to go wrong next.

There are few things more enjoyable for most of us than eating the foods that we love. Food should be enjoyed! However, for the next few pages, I would like you to forget about the taste of food. I would like to help you to understand that the foods that you eat are a critical *investment* in your health.

First and foremost, food is a source of the raw materials that you need to build a strong, healthy body. *Those raw materials are especially important during the rest periods after an exercise investment.* It is during this time that your body is rebuilding to become stronger. You just can't build a great body with jelly doughnuts and Cheetos.

DIFFERENT HOMES, DIFFERENT MATERIALS

All dream homes are different. They require different raw materials. Though every home requires certain basics, like lumber for the walls and wires for the electrical system, the *quantity* and *type* of materials will vary greatly depending on what you are building. The architect draws the plans before the builder orders the materials. You need a plan before you purchase the amount and types of the building blocks that you will need.

Similarly, in designing and building your "dream body," you are going to need to know what you want to create. All bodies need certain foods. I will provide some general guidelines on what to eat in this chapter. However, if you are a 105-pound, thirty-year-old female executive and your husband is an overweight fifty-year-old construction superintendent, both of you cannot eat the same way for optimal health. No two people should eat the same diet.

The problem with fad diets, the old "food pyramid," and other traditional approaches to diet is that they are not tailored to the individual. They do not take into account the differences in the *amount* of food or the *kinds* of food that are needed between individuals. In the area of nutrition, one size does not fit all.

In addition, *food preferences* must be taken into account. Anyone can write a good nutritional plan on paper. It is easy for a registered dietician to calculate the number of calories a person should eat and then balance those calories among healthy food groups from a book. But if the food is unacceptable to the individual, it just won't work! This is why generalized nutritional approaches fail. This is one value of a concierge physician: he can help you tailor a program to meet your likes as well as your needs.

A MOVE TOWARD INDIVIDUALIZING NUTRITION

Nutrition must also be coordinated with the *volume* and *intensity* of your exercise investments. Even the U.S. government has recognized this fact. Current nutritional guidelines put forth by the U.S. Department of Agriculture have been modified to address differences in levels of physical activity. Instead of recommending that every American follow the same "food pyramid," they now have twelve different pyramids to choose from.

If you go to the USDA food pyramid Web site (www.mypyramid. gov), you will find a new, interactive program. Before any nutritional information is dispensed, you will have to enter your age, sex, and *level of activity*. Programs like these are a good step toward individualizing your dietary plan.

As a way of providing a base of nutritional knowledge, I am going to address two topics in this chapter. The first topic is *weight loss*. The second is the *nutritional value* or the quality of the foods that you eat. The rest will be up to you and your doctor.

WEIGHT LOSS

"Oh My God, What Is That?"

Over the past fifteen years, I have counseled literally thousands of people who have wanted to lose weight. These people were universally frustrated. Some of them were legitimately confused. Many were just looking for a "quick fix."

There is a lot of conflicting information out there regarding diets. There is also a lot of voodoo dispensed as "science." What is a fad diet? What is a legitimate diet? What about low-carb diets? Or the Zone diet? Adding to the confusion over legitimacy is the fact that most diet books are authored by an M.D. or a Ph.D. Which doctor is real? Which doctor is a witch doctor? It is not always easy for the layperson to tell.

Over the years, I've used various strategies to teach my patients about weight loss. I have tried to help them understand the subject of body composition. I have tried using science. I've tried using humor. I've tried to be supportive. I've tried "tough love." Yet most of these things have not worked. My words have often been ineffective.

Finally, I stumbled onto a wonderful teaching tool for weight loss. It works because most of us are *visual learners*. It cost me only $80. This remarkable tool is a replica of a pound of body fat. It sits in my examining room on a table. When people take a look at that pound of fat, they usually say, "Oh my God, what is that?"

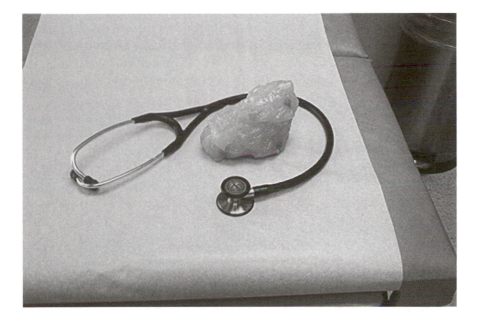

If I have people who are trying to lose weight, I put that pound of fat in their hands. I let them hold it and feel it. I don't do this to be cruel. I want them to understand what a Krispy Kreme doughnut morphs into after a few hours in their digestive system. I want them to know how their body stores excess energy. I want them to *see* and *feel* how excess calories and junk food are recorded in their liability column.

I then explain to my patient that each pound of fat is nothing more than a source of stored fuel. It is excess energy that their body never needed. To burn just 1 pound of fat, they will need to burn 3,500 calories doing exercise.

Alternatively, to lose that fat, they could eat fewer calories to create a *calorie deficit*. I tell my patients that if they were to spend an hour on the treadmill or the exercise bike, they would only burn about 350 calories. I do the math with them. *To burn just 1 pound of fat, they would need to spend 10 hours on that treadmill.* Unless they cut back on their calories, the amount of exercise needed to lose weight is staggering.

I explain how tight nature is with its accounting. Most people are amazed. I then explain that a typical candy bar, which is often described by my patients as "just a little slip in their diet," contains 250–350 calories. If they spend 45 minutes to an hour on the treadmill and then eat that candy bar, they have just wiped out their exercise investment. This is pretty humbling. But again, these are nature's laws, not mine. They reflect simple Darwinian natural selection. Before food was so plentiful, it was advantageous for our ancestors to be able to store fuel very efficiently and to hang on to those stored calories for times of need. Now, in our present world where food is so abundant, this genetic trait is a liability. We therefore have to use our brains to adapt to new conditions if we are to survive.

Understanding the number of calories contained within a pound of fat explains why so many people say, "I don't understand it. I eat pretty well. I exercise, but I still can't lose weight." The problem is that they just don't understand the numbers. They just don't understand that eating "pretty well" will not get them where they want to be, especially if by pretty well they are comparing their diet to the average American diet, which is horrible.

What Is a Calorie?

The term "calorie" has no tangible meaning for most people. A calorie is a scientific term. It is a unit of measure of energy in the metric system. A calorie is defined as the amount of energy required to raise the temperature of 1 gram of water by 1°Celsius. This is a true calorie, sometimes called a "small calorie." When discussing nutrition, a calorie actually represents a kilocalorie, or 1,000 calories. You see, this definition just doesn't reach people where they live. We don't think in terms of metric units of energy in our daily lives. The term calorie just doesn't hit us like the visual of that pound of fat!

After they've held that pound of fat in their hands, I measure my patient's body composition. When they realize that they are carrying 30 extra pounds of body fat, they are shocked. They will point at the pound of fat and say, "I have thirty of those ugly things in my body!" It is at this point that they have an understanding of and appreciation for the impact of excess body fat on their health. Now I am communicating in a language that they can understand. It becomes a teachable moment. They suddenly realize that this excess body fat is *their* problem. It will be up to *them* to change it.

This is not trickery. It is not a scare tactic. It is a visual learning tool. Most of us are visual learners. Unless we see something, we just don't get it. This simple model allows nonmedical people to see what body fat actually looks like. When doctors go into the operating room they see real body fat all the time. When a heart surgeon makes an incision on an overweight person during a bypass operation, he cuts through globs of yellow fat. When a radiologist views the CT scan of an obese person, the fat is clearly visible under the skin and surrounding the abdominal organs. But the average person never sees what body fat really looks like. The enemy is hidden in an increased dress size or belt notch. Looking at a pound of fat is one of those "Aha!" moments. This is why I have included the photo in this book for you.

Healthy Tissue

To contrast that pound of fat, I have another visual tool in my office. It is a replica of a pound of muscle. People are often told that "muscle weighs more than fat." What they really mean is that it is more dense than fat. However, they often really don't understand this concept until they see the two next models to each other. Though both models weigh 1 pound, the pound of fat is bigger. It takes up more volume than a pound of muscle.

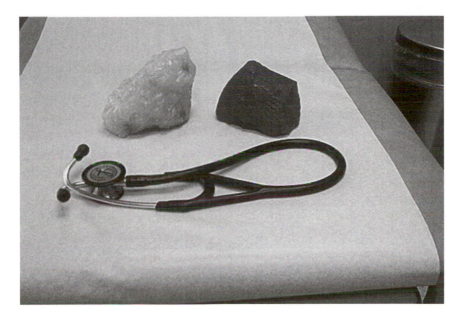

After showing them that pound of muscle, I explain why this kind of healthy tissue is an asset. Unlike fat, muscle propels you. Lean muscle burns energy, even at rest. It increases your metabolism, or the number of calories that your body burns. Therefore, by increasing the amount of lean muscle in your body, you will burn more calories at rest and during exercise, hence helping you to stay lean and reduce your body fat. Fat, on the other hand, just sits there. It takes very little energy to maintain fat. It is a drain on your health assets.

In addition, muscle tissue requires quality nutrients to sustain. Muscle requires healthy building blocks from your diet. Fat does not.

For women who cringe when I suggest that they create more muscle, I explain that they will not look like body builders with more lean muscle. Instead, if they replace that bulkier fat with leaner tissue, they will be smaller. They will look healthier and more defined. They will also be stronger. They will reduce their risk of cancer. They will stay thin and lean more easily, and they will look good.

There is absolutely nothing wrong with using your desire to look better or to be sexier as a motivational tool. Use whatever motivates you! Even if vanity is your primary driving force, you will get the health benefits of becoming leaner if you begin to replace excess body fat with muscle.

The Liability of Excess Body Fat

There are few things that will depreciate your body faster than an excess of body fat. The only other factor that has such a detrimental impact on health is a sedentary lifestyle. The combination of the two, being overweight and sedentary, is a recipe for personal bankruptcy. Interestingly, despite our great financial wealth in this country, a baby born in the United States will live, on average, seventy-eight years. Our life expectancy ranks only forty-second in the world, down from eleventh twenty years ago; this, despite the fact that we have the most advanced medical technology available on the planet. Clearly, our epidemic of obesity and a sedentary lifestyle is having a terribly detrimental impact on our bodies.

Being overweight alone is associated with a myriad of diseases that slowly destroys your most precious asset. These problems are well known to most people. They include heart disease, stroke, diabetes, breast cancer, ovarian cancer, premature arthritis of the knees and hips, back problems, and depression. If this were not enough, excess body fat eats away at people psychologically. When appearance suffers, self-esteem suffers. With a loss of self-esteem and feeling good inside your skin comes a loss of sexual appetite. Being overweight is like an unhealthy house of cards.

The pressing question for most people is how to get rid of that excess body fat. How do you reduce your health liabilities? What about those fad diets? Even if they are unhealthy in the short run, should you try a fad diet to get the weight off quickly? Should you eat poorly in the beginning and eat healthier later?

The Great Diet Debate

A few years ago, I was asked to debate a well-known cardiologist who had been recommending the Atkins diet for his heart patients. A small advertisement was put in the newspapers by the promoters of the event. The next morning, the venue had to be changed. Over 300 people had called to reserve their place in the auditorium. The venue was changed twice again due to a huge demand. On the evening of the debate at the Westin La Paloma Hotel, the parking lot had to be closed. It was filled to capacity. As I walked into the auditorium, I was met by a standing-room-only crowd of 1,200 people. There were many doctors in the audience, some of whom were actually on the Atkins diet themselves. There were TV crews and newspaper reporters. Everyone had come to "hear the truth" about low-carb diets and decide for themselves about the merits of the Atkins diet.

The winner was to be judged by the public using an applause meter at the end of the debate. I presented scientific study after study documenting the problems with a high-fat, nutrient-poor diet. I explained that after thirty-five years of public use, not a single study had been conducted to see if the Atkins diet produced any sustained weight loss. Put simply, there was no scientific evidence for the efficacy or safety of the diet. I had three assistants walk out on stage and pour 83 pounds of animal fat into a large transparent container. This is the average amount of animal fat consumed in one year by a person on the Atkins diet. Despite all the data and my theatrics, only half of the audience was convinced. The following morning, the front page of the *Arizona Daily Star* read, "Diet Debate Ends in a Draw."

Interestingly, I would later learn that some of the audience perceived me as "mean." During the debate, I showed a slide of Dr. Atkins' Web site, demonstrating that he sold cheesecake, pancake mix, and untested formulas to cure everything from the common cold to PMS. I pointed out that Dr. Atkins' sales and marketing machine met the congressional definition for quackery. None of his theories or products had been tested to prove their claims. Instead of being outraged that a cardiologist would behave in such an irresponsible manner, some in the audience turned against me for pointing out that this emperor had no clothes. It was a fascinating study in human nature. For many in the audience on the Atkins diet, it was as if I were criticizing their personal religion. I was somehow trampling on sacred ground and had no right to legitimately question Atkins' claims.

A year after the debate, the *New England Journal of Medicine* published the first controlled study on the Atkins diet. After assigning people to a year on the Atkins diet versus a year on a conventional low-fat diet, the results were virtually the same. *People on the Atkins diet were no more successful at weight loss than those on a low-fat diet.* Regardless of any health risks of the Atkins diet, it just doesn't work. It is not a good investment strategy. It will not reduce your fat liabilities in the long run. It is not a "jump start" and it will not help you get to a goal of fat loss any faster.

The Atkins diet, like other "low-carb diets," should be more accurately termed a "high-fat diet." If you analyze the composition of foods on this "low-carb diet," you will find that 60–70 percent of calories come from animal fat. Fat is not an optimal building block for your body. It does not provide vital building blocks after exercise. Atkins himself realized that his diet lacked many vital nutrients that come from fruits and vegetables. He responded to this legitimate criticism by selling dozens of "vita-nutrients" that could be purchased in stores and on his Web site. He made millions doing this. However, people are finally beginning to realize that this approach does not work. The low-carb diet craze is finally coming to an end. Atkins Nutritionals Inc. filed for bankruptcy in August 2005.

Calorie Accounting 101

You may wonder why I am so confident that fad diets are such a poor investment strategy. Why isn't there a quick fix? Isn't it okay to accelerate a weight loss and then eat for health later? Rule number 1: *You can't burn fat quickly*! You may be able to "lose weight" quickly, in the form of water weight, but that will do nothing for your health and appearance and will only dehydrate you.

No matter what anyone tells you, you can't lose 5 pounds of fat in a week, at least not without an enormous amount of exercise.

Let's do the math and see what would be required to burn five pounds of fat in a week, using what we know about the 3,500 calories contained in that ugly pound of fat:

- Five pounds of fat contains $5 \times 3,500$ calories/per pound of fat, which is equal to 17,500 calories. This is the calorie deficit that you would need to create over a seven-day period to lose those 5 pounds of fat. You would literally need to eat 17,500 *fewer* calories per week than you burn over a week.
- If you spread this 17,500-calorie deficit over seven days, you would need a 2,500-calorie deficit each day.
- Let's say you eat only 1,000 calories per day on a fad diet. This isn't many calories. If you have a reasonable metabolism, you may burn 2,000 calories per day. This would create only a 1,000-calorie per day deficit, not the necessary 2,500 calories.
- A 1000-calorie deficit for seven days is equal to a **7,000-calorie** deficit for the week. This is far from the 17,500-calorie per week deficit needed to lose 5 pounds of fat!

What if you add in "a little exercise"? Could you lose 5 pounds of fat in a week on a fad diet with moderate exercise? If you do the math, you would need to burn an additional 10,500 calories in exercise per week to lose those 5 pounds of fat. Burning calories at a rate of 350 per hour, you would literally need to spend 30 hours per week on the treadmill and eat only 1,000 calories per day to lose 5 pounds of body fat in one week! Check my math:

- Exercise on the treadmill is equal to 350 calories burned per hour. 10,500 calories divided by 350 calories burned per hour is equal to 30 hours of exercise per week.
- 30 hours of exercise per week divided by 7 days is equal to 4.3 hours of exercise per day.

So, if you limit your food intake to 1,000 calories per day and walk on a treadmill for 4 hours per day, you will lose 5 pounds of fat over the next week. I can assure you that most people on the Atkins diet eat more than 1,000 calories per day. When people claim that they lost 5 pounds in their first week on a fad diet, they lost water, not body fat.

The Truth Is in the Numbers

Remember, just as in financial investing, the truth about your health is in the numbers. There is no magic when it comes to fat loss. The numbers tell the real story, not the seller of a fad diet. The reason that I have taken you through this painful arithmetic exercise is so that you trust what I am saying is true. You can verify the numbers for yourself.

These numbers explain why most experts suggest that you try to lose only 1 pound of fat per week. Losing a pound of fat per week still takes work. It requires a 500-calorie per day deficit. If you spend about 45 minutes on the treadmill every day and cut 200 calories from your diet, you will create that 500-calorie per day deficit. A 500-calorie per day deficit for seven days will give you the 3,500-calorie deficit needed to lose that pound of fat in a week.

The point is that a calorie is a calorie. It is a unit of energy. No matter what the diet author claims, calories don't vanish into thin air if you eat some specific combination of foods. This is just wishful thinking. If you are going to limit your calories to lose body fat, why not eat *quality calories*? Why would you want to eat 70 percent of your calories from animal fat in order to lose body water? It makes no sense. Eating more fat does not magically burn fat. If you are exercising while you diet, it is especially unwise to eat a high-fat, low-carb diet. This kind of diet simply does not provide the nutrients you need to fuel growing muscle and healthy tissue. You need the nutrients contained within fruits and vegetables. You also need complex carbohydrates, which are the primary fuel for muscle contraction.

What about the Carbs?

Just a word on carbohydrates. Contrary to popular belief, carbs do not make you fat, provided that they are not consumed in excess. If you eat three servings of pasta in a sitting or consume half a loaf of bread, you will ingest a lot of excess calories. Any consumption of excess calories will be stored as body fat, whether those calories come in the form of fats, proteins, or carbohydrates.

In my experience, many people who are on a "low-fat" craze don't understand this fact. They start eating carbohydrates and they can't stop themselves. I had a nurse in my practice, for example, who told me that she ate nonfat cookies in an attempt to satisfy her cravings and lose weight. When I asked how many cookies she ate, she replied, "The whole box!" Though this may sound absurd, I've had many people tell me that they sit down and eat huge quantities of complex carbohydrates. They'll eat an entire bag of "baked" potato chips, three servings of spaghetti, or an entire nonfat coffee cake.

Complex carbohydrates are the primary fuel for the body during exercise. Complex carbohydrates are chains of small sugar molecules linked together. When you eat complex carbohydrates, they are stored in muscle in the form of glycogen for future exercise. Complex carbohydrates include potatoes, rice, beans, pasta, bread, fruits, and vegetables. The more you exercise, the more complex carbohydrates you will need to fuel your body.

The other misconception about carbohydrates comes when people lump simple sugars into the category of carbohydrates. Though simple sugars are technically a carbohydrate, high-sugar foods are calorie-dense and contain a lot of calories per unit volume.

When I did the diet debate, the cardiologist called doughnuts "carbohydrates." Actually, the bulk of calories in doughnuts does not come from the flour. If you don't believe me, read the nutritional label on a box of doughnuts. Most of the calories in a doughnut come from the fat and sugar. Only about 25 percent of the calories come from the complex carbohydrate we call flour.

The amount of carbohydrates you should eat will depend on how much you exercise. Each gram of carbohydrate contains only 4 calories. Each gram of fat contains 9 calories.

The Three-Day Diet Log

The best way to really know what you are currently eating is to write down every morsel of food that you put in your mouth over a three- to five-day period. To get a sense of when and where you overeat, it may be wise to do your diet log on both weekdays and weekends. The results of this exercise are often very surprising to the eater. Many of us eat subconsciously. We forget what we snack on during the day. We may eat out of stress or out of reflex. We are not always aware of just *how much* we eat or *what* we eat. The diet log is like holding up a mirror. It gives us objective information. It uncovers unhealthy behavior patterns so that we can make change.

Once I have reviewed a three-day diet log, I can begin to see where the problems lie for my patient. I not only see where their excess calories come from, I can also look at their nutritional status. I can see if they are getting the vital nutrients they need to invest in their most precious asset.

Many people have specific behavioral patterns of poor eating that undo their goals. Some people are able to eat well during the day. At night, after a cocktail, or in front of the TV, their resolve weakens. They may starve themselves during the day, skipping breakfast or lunch, and then become ravenous in the evening. Once they start bingeing they can't stop. Others dine out frequently and unknowingly eat foods with hidden calories. They'll order fish, which is healthy, covered in a butter cream sauce. Others just snack all day and never eat real meals. Reviewing your diet log with your doctor can help you identify where your specific problems lie.

Making Change

Even if you know that you are not eating well, you may not be able to give up your bad habits so easily. We all have bad habits. The reason that we repeat bad habits is that they do something for us. People drink too much alcohol because they think it is fun. They can temporarily escape from the multitude of stresses that affect their daily lives. People smoke for similar reasons. We overeat because it provides us with momentary pleasure. No one is immune from bad habits. It is only a matter of degree.

The only way that I can convince you to consider changing a self-destructive habit like overeating is if I am able to offer you something better to replace the habit that you are currently engaged in. You may have seen a popular saying on a button that reads, "Nothing tastes as good as thin feels." This saying gets to my point. Food is fun. But looking and feeling better is *more* fun than being fat.

To change a bad investment strategy like eating poorly, there has to be something in it for you. To find the trade-off, find out what makes you tick. Above all, be honest with yourself. You don't have to tell anyone else about your motivation if you don't want to. Find out *why* you want to lose excess body fat. If it is vanity, admit it to yourself. Use it. If it is a recent heart attack or fear of poor health, use your fear to motivate you.

I once had a thirty-year-old woman walk into my office and say, "This may sound silly, but I used to look great on the beach in a thong bikini. I want to look great in a thong again." My response? "Great! Have at it." This is *your* goal. If you are a fifty-five-year-old bank president who just had his first heart attack and you want to see your grandchildren grow, use your fear of premature death as your motivation. Is that Twinkie in the cupboard really worth more than a trip to Disneyland with your grandson? You decide. Invest accordingly.

Behavioral science has attempted to examine why it is that we don't always do what is in our best interests. In truth what we understand about behavior, our motivations, and the way that our brains work is far behind the rest of medical science. What we are left with at the moment are limited behavior theories. One of the most popular models is the Stages of Change model of behavior. The various stages we go through in giving up destructive behaviors are listed below:

1. Precontemplation (Not yet acknowledging that we have a problem or behavior that needs to be changed. This is characterized by denial or ambivalence—a battle over wanting to stop a destructive behavior and continuing the behavior.)
2. Contemplation (We acknowledge that there is a problem, but we are not ready to make a change.)
3. Preparation (We begin thinking about making a change but have no plan of action.)
4. Action (We take steps to change our behavior.)
5. Relapse (We resume our prior self-destructive behavior.)

Most people do not succeed in changing undesirable behaviors with the first try. They often relapse before they ultimately succeed. This observed pattern is certainly seen in people who attempt to lose weight. But there is nothing in this behavior model that tells us about the mechanism of behavior. For example, this certainly does not address our genetic drive to eat! It is purely observational. The take-home message is that if you fail at healthy eating initially, or if you relapse, just try again until you get it right!

Dr. Tammy Basford, the Director of Family Medicine at the University of Arizona, puts it this way: "The current behavioral techniques that we use to teach patients about healthier lifestyles are very blunt instruments. They are not tailored to the individual. We cannot approach everyone the same way. AA is a great model for white, middle-class businessmen with alcohol problems, but it fails miserably for other groups of people." Tammy's comments are so true. The best ally that you can have is a physician who can explore what motivates you personally to change. He can use your unique motivational triggers along with his clinical expertise to help keep you focused to reach your goals.

A doctor who has time to get to know you has a better shot at effectively practicing the *art of medicine*, which involves tailoring science to the individual. You just can't address a behavioral problem like poor eating in a 12-minute office visit.

BEYOND WEIGHT LOSS: THE SUBJECT OF NUTRITION

In the last chapter on exercise, I told you that good nutrition is especially important during rest periods. After you've made an investment of exercise, your body requires the necessary building blocks to become stronger. Though you may not be actively exercising during this rest period, your body is very active in retooling to make you stronger. This concept of fueling your body optimally may not sound very exciting, but it can be. Just think of it like building wealth!

When you were first exposed to the concept of saving money to build wealth, it was probably not very exciting; especially when you were young. Who wants to save money when you can get that immediate gratification from spending above your means? However, after a little life experience squandering some cash, you soon realized that short-term gain could result in long-term pain. You began to adjust your thinking.

With maturity, the knowledge that you can use some of your capital for investing to make your money grow for the future is exciting. When you mature and understand that you can use your capital to buy freedom, your motivation further increases.

The purpose of investing in your diet is to buy freedom from disease and disability in your life. Sure you want to splurge and throw caution to the wind every once in a while. Feasts are fun. But more importantly, you want to be vibrant. You want a great sex life. You want to feel great and look great. You want to live longer. The more that you invest in good eating habits on a consistent basis, the greater freedom you will create in your life.

Nutrient-Rich vs. Calorie-Dense Foods

Like the exercise curve that I showed you in the previous chapter, I am going to share some important fundamental concepts that will help you eat better. This will get you started before you have a chance to analyze your own situation more carefully with your doctor. In my view, the two most important nutritional concepts are (1) calorie density and (2) nutrient-to-calorie ratio.

The reason that so many people are overweight in this country is that they eat too many *calorie-dense foods*. By this I mean that they eat foods that have many calories packed into a very small volume. These foods typically contain a lot of fat and sugar. They are also nutrient-poor. An example of a calorie-dense food is a chocolate truffle. This tasty little morsel is only the size of a marble. However, it contains 106 calories. It is composed of 8.5 grams of sugar, 8.8 grams of fat, and only 1.8 grams of protein. It is made with whipping cream, chocolate, butter, liqueur, almonds, and sugar. Apart from the almonds, there are few nutrients in a truffle. Eat lots of these little jewels and you will add to your liability column.

Like you, I've been through my share of boring checkout lines at the grocery store. There isn't much to do. I often find myself people watching. I've yet to see an overweight person ask the bag boy to help them with massive quantities of fresh corn, tomatoes, chicken breasts, whole grains, and apples. What I usually see instead are bags of Oreo cookies, chips and dip, rich salad dressings, ground hamburger meat, ice cream, and other food "luxuries." The reason for this observation is clear. It is much harder to become fat by eating healthier foods than it is by eating junk. Healthy foods are not as calorie-dense as junk foods.

As I pointed out earlier, part of the problem of obesity in our country is due to the fact that food is so readily available; we don't have to hunt and gather like our ancestors did. However, this statement is only part of the story. If we ate larger quantities of *healthier* foods and remained active, we would not have such a problem with obesity in our country.

It is the quality of "foods" that we consume, along with a sedentary lifestyle, that has created the problem.

How about eating just three of those Oreo Cookies from the bag, as if that were an easy trick! Oreo cookies are not what I would consider food. Oreos are the result of a chemistry experiment. Three Oreos contain the following nutritional profile: Calories = 160; Total fat = 7grams; Total sugar = 13 grams; Nutrients = Almost 0!

It's not just that we have too much food available to us. It is that the food that is available in abundance barely resembles food—it is nutrient-poor.

The Key to Nutritious Investing: Watching Your Nutrient-to-Calorie Ratio

The key to nutritional investing is to understand a simple concept called the *nutrient-to-calorie ratio*. The nutrient-to-calorie ratio looks at the number of nutrients per calorie contained within a given food. The higher the ratio, the more nutritious the food; the lower the ratio, the poorer the quality of the food.

You should try to eat foods that have a lot of good nutrients packed into each calorie of food that you eat. Since you can only eat so many calories before starting to store the excess as fat, you want to allocate your calories wisely.

Managing a calorie budget is like managing money. You only have so much money to invest. In investing, you pick a group of stocks that have the most value-to-cost ratio. If you choose a bunch of poor performers in your portfolio, you are not going to grow capital. Likewise, if your calories are used up on nutrient-poor foods, your health portfolio declines in value.

Foods that contain significant amounts of one or more nutrients in relation to the number of calories they contain are called "nutrient-dense." Examples of nutrient-dense foods are lean meats, nonfat dairy products, and even eggs. The kind of nutrients found in these nutrient-dense foods include a high quality of protein, iron, zinc, riboflavin, niacin, and vitamins B6 and B12. You see, I'm not trying to turn you into a vegetarian. If you are a vegetarian, great. But if not, there is nothing wrong with a 4-ounce cut of lean filet mignon. It has a similar nutrient-to-calorie ratio as a chicken breast. It is a great nutritional investment, especially if you like the taste of red meat.

If you like red meat, just make sure that you limit the portion sizes. This is where most people get into trouble. Four ounces of steak is about the size of a deck of cards. A healthy serving of red meat is not that 12- or 16-ounce steak that you pay $30 for at your local steak house. Remember, too much of any food is converted into health liabilities.

Other foods with a high nutrient-to-calorie ratio include colored fruits and vegetables, seafood, whole grains, beans, and nuts. This is why your mother made you hold your nose and eat your veggies! She knew that these foods were good for you. Provided you don't use a lot of rich salad dressing, you can get a lot of nutrients from vegetables with very few calories. Fruits like strawberries are another source of excellent nutrients with relatively few calories. They taste great too! To end on an up note, here's a little good news on the good-tasting food front. Over the past year, chocolate and coffee have both shown some very real health benefits in legitimate studies. Coffee contains a great deal of antioxidants. Dark chocolate, in small quantities equivalent to about one and one-half Hershey's kisses per day, can lower blood pressure.

Healthy Eating Plans

Though I do not endorse any diet plan per se, there are several healthy eating plans that you may want to consider as starting resources. All of these plans can be easily investigated on the Internet.

- *My Pyramid*: Though the food pyramid has gotten a bad rap, there is nothing wrong with it. As I mentioned, it has been revamped and individualized to sex, age, and activity level. You might try looking at the new food pyramid, renamed My Food Pyramid. The information is free.
- *The Mediterranean Diet*: One of the most popular forms of "healthier eating" is the Mediterranean diet. It contains many tasty, nutrient-dense foods. It is sexier than the food pyramid. It conjures up images of dining in Greece while overlooking the sea. Imagine having a glass of red wine and dining on a piece of fresh seafood, some veggies sautéed in olive oil, and fruit for dessert. Now that sounds a lot more appealing than a salad bar for many people! Olive oil and nuts are substituted for unhealthier saturated fats in this diet. The only issue is that more than half of the calories come from monounsaturated fats, primarily the olive oil. With a little modification, it can be a very healthy eating plan.
- *The DASH Diet*: This diet has been extensively studied and scientifically proven to lower blood pressure and cholesterol and meet all of the criteria

for nutrient-rich eating. It has been endorsed by the American Heart Association. It is rich in fruits and vegetables, combined with nonfat dairy products. It is extremely healthy, although a little spartan for meat lovers. I frequently use this diet for those people who have mild high blood pressure and want to try to avoid taking medications. The National Heart, Blood and Lung Institute offers a book on the DASH diet for $3.50. Just type in DASH diet on the Internet for more information.

- *Weight Watchers*: Like the revamped Food Pyramid, this is not your mother's Weight Watchers. The plan is inexpensive. It is based on sound nutritional principles. There are lots of interesting and tasty recipes provided by the company. For those who want a support group atmosphere, the company offers inexpensive meetings and computer-based resources. What I like about Weight Watchers is that you can get good nutritional information without being hooked on buying a lot of products.

Planning for an Occasional Binge

Life without parties is not a rich life. You should plan those nights when you are going to pull out all the stops. If you want to remain in calorie balance while indulging in an occasional binge, do what I do. Skip lunch that day and have some fun. If you normally eat 700 calories for lunch, just tack those calories on at dinner time. The next day you won't feel quite so terrible. It won't really affect your liability column.

When you are trying to solidify new habits, I would recommend that you avoid doing too much binge eating. Try to wait until you've actually reached your goal and solidified new behaviors before you leap off the wagon. Otherwise, you are likely to lapse back into your old, self-destructive patterns. Think of food indulgences the way that you think of financial indulgences, like vacations or a new toy. Use them as a treat. Use them sparingly, until you have the base of health-wealth that you desire.

Your Internal Calorie Counter

If you've ever tried to count calories, you know that it is very difficult to do so accurately. It is cumbersome and time-consuming to measure your food. Fortunately it is not necessary, because you have a built-in calorie counter. This built-in calorie counter is called your appetite. The problem is that many people have forgotten how to use it.

When you are eating and you begin to feel full, stop eating. Take this advice literally: when you are full, *do not eat one extra bite*. You are done. It's fine to leave food on your plate. It's fine to leave a restaurant with food on the table. If you don't want to do this, take the leftovers home in a doggie bag. Just don't eat when you are not hungry.

If fat loss is your goal, being a little hungry is a necessary component of being in a negative calorie balance. There is no way to lose fat and not be just a little hungry all the time. If you seem to crave more food while trying to lose weight, don't think of that feeling as hunger but as the sensation of losing weight—that your plan is actually working!

Many people are so used to overeating that they have temporarily blunted their awareness of that feeling of fullness. They eat for sport. In my observations of many patients, a sense of normal fullness begins to return after people become more active. They become more in tune with their body as they begin to listen to their appetite. They develop greater "body awareness."

Nutritional Investing

So what are the essential guidelines for investing in your nutrition? Keep it simple:

1. Avoid calorie-dense foods that add more pounds of fat to your liability column.
2. Consume foods that have a high nutrient-to-calorie ratio.
3. Stop eating when you are full. Listen to your body.
4. If you are trying to lose body fat, be a little hungry all the time.

If you can do these simple things, your body composition and your health will improve significantly. If you use these concepts combined with a tailor-made nutritional program from your doctor, you will be well on your way to a leaner, stronger, and healthier body.

CHAPTER 8

What's Wrong with Concierge Medicine?

Concierge medicine has its share of critics. Some have even described it as "unethical." The basic concern centers on the fear that concierge medicine will lead to a three-tiered healthcare system. It is argued that those at the top of the economic food chain will have unlimited access to good healthcare, while the poor will continue to use ERs and free clinics. The middle class will remain mired in a system of HMOs, PPOs, and a failing Medicare program.

I will be the first to acknowledge that concierge medicine will do little to solve many of the most pressing healthcare problems in this country. As I pointed out earlier, concierge medicine is nothing more than a form of private medicine, which has been around for as long as doctors have accepted fees directly from their patients. Private medical practices were never started as a way to solve our national healthcare problems, any more than private law firms were created to solve the problems of those who cannot afford expert legal counsel.

Concierge medicine is a patient-driven movement that is evolving to meet the needs of those who are fed up with our present incompetent system. With the exception of pro-bono work that is done by concierge doctors, it is limited to those with middle- and upper-class incomes.

THE BASIC CONTROVERSY

From the *Arizona Daily Star* to *The New York Times*, most articles that have been written on concierge medicine have followed a similar format. The story usually begins with a patient who is able to immediately access his doctor. The doctor solves a serious medical problem. The patient is delighted. The doctor is content with his new professional life. Everybody goes home happy.

Next, a critic from an academic medical center is quoted. He describes concierge medicine as "unethical" or, at best, "mercenary." A counter argument is made by either a concierge doctor or other physician who responds in a logical and politically correct manner. This doctor reminds us that we live in a free country. Unless we are willing to tell people how to spend their money in other areas of their lives, there is nothing wrong with concierge medicine. To criticize concierge medicine is to criticize the American way. So the debate goes.

In a recent article in *Managed Care* magazine, Dr. Jay Jacobson, a professor of internal medicine at the University of Utah's School of Medicine, presented the ethicists' position as follows: "*It's unprofessional. If doctors feel too pressed by the current insurance system to treat patients properly, then perhaps they should push for a change in the system rather than for a practice model that simply makes their own lives simpler and makes individual doctors more successful but misses the mark on physicians' collective goal: 'To provide more and better care for **more** [emphasis added] people [italics mine].'*"

Presenting the opposing view favoring concierge medicine was the past President of the AMA, Dr. Yank Coble. Dr. Coble responded, "*Concierge medicine is not an appropriate term. Retainer Medicine is more accurate. First, patients are pushing the trend with a desire to have easier access, for longer periods, to the physician of their choice—rather than picking a name off a network list* [italics mine]." Dr. Coble went on to say, "*No one hesitates to pay a lawyer or accountant a retainer. That's a widely accepted business model for professionals—as well as a solid reason to believe that today's medical novelty may well become tomorrow's widely copied health care norm* [italics mine]."

When I opened the first concierge practice in the state of Arizona seven years ago, I experienced the same criticisms as those leveled by Dr. Jacobson. I was called selfish and unethical. The following quote from a University of Arizona professor appeared on the front page of the *Arizona Daily Star*: "*This is boutique medicine at its mercenary worst* [italics mine]."

I don't take this criticism personally. This is politics. It sells newspaper copies. Going back to our good friend Dr. Welby, nobody ever criticized Marcus for delivering compassionate, comprehensive medical care on a fee-for-service basis. However, comments like this don't address the *real* ethical issues facing concierge medicine. Furthermore, if we are going to talk about the medical ethics of concierge medicine and its potential impact on the system, we need to look at the ethics of the entire healthcare system.

THE ETHICS OF OUR PRESENT HEALTHCARE SYSTEM

It is important to pause for a moment and consider carefully what Dr. Jacobson said in the quotation above. The implication is that it is somehow nobler for doctors to care for large numbers of patients in our current assembly-line healthcare delivery system than to focus their efforts on quality care for fewer patients. Think about this position for a moment. Is it more "ethical" to spend 8–12 minutes delivering hurried, superficial care to thirty patients per day on an HMO plan than it is to take 20 to 30 minutes with fifteen patients and provide more compressive care? If so, what is more ethical about it?

More importantly, is it "ethical" for a doctor to sign an HMO contract in the first place? When a doctor contracts with an HMO, he agrees to play by their rules. He knows that the medical care that he recommends to his patients may be *denied* by the HMO. He knows that he may have to cut corners in exchange for the financial benefit of receiving a large number of patients that will be delivered by the HMO. He knows that his medical judgment may be overridden by an administrator for the company. In a very real sense, he becomes the *financial advocate* of the HMO by signing the contract. He is no longer just a patient advocate. One of the fundamental axioms passed on by Hippocrates was *Primum non nocere—Above all do no harm.* Is it ethical for a physician to sign a contract, knowing that this may harm a patient, provided that it pays the doctor's mortgage?

Like any business that sells stock to the public, the HMO has a fiscal and fiduciary responsibility to its shareholders. The for-profit HMO is in business for the sole purpose of turning a profit. The purpose of the HMO is to grow capital for its investors. This is not a "medical model"; it is a "business model."

As I will explain later, the only way for an HMO to turn a profit for its stockholders is to *ration* care to patients. In this model of medical delivery, the person who decides how care is to be rationed is not your doctor; it is an executive in your HMO. Is it "ethical" for a doctor to sign a contract with an HMO, agreeing to ration care for thirty patients every day, when he is aware that such arrangements have caused serious harm and even death to patients?

I have no trouble with capitalism or Wall Street. I support it. Businesses must be profitable to survive. People have every right to grow their wealth and companies have the right and responsibility to turn a profit. This is how capitalism operates. However, I don't believe that the large fast-food corporate model works in caring for patients. In my view, the current system is not ethical. Ironically, though it is concierge physicians who are called "mercenary," it is the HMO that is explicitly mercenary.

MY JOURNEY INTO CONCIERGE MEDICINE

I have personally lived through the process of trying to change our broken healthcare system. I continue to work for change. But now I do it in a different manner. I am working to create a viable alternative as opposed to battling our broken system. I was a leader in the medical community. I was a strong advocate for reform. Shortly after going into medical practice, I tried to *"push for a change in the system,"* as Dr. Jacobson suggested. I was the Chief of Medicine at a 400-bed community hospital. I formed and personally funded an organization called the Tucson Alliance for Medical Excellence in an attempt to improve the healthcare in my HMO-dominated city.

Like most doctors, I went into medicine with the noblest of intentions. I understood nothing about the *business* of medicine. I believed that if I simply concentrated on doing the best that I could with each patient, the rest would fall into place. I assumed that my skills would be respected by insurance carriers who needed me to serve their members. To put it kindly, I was naïve. In the vernacular, I was wet behind the ears.

Before getting a business education in the real-world practice of medicine, I did not understand the magnitude of the financial and political forces that would dominate the quality of the medicine that I could deliver. I did not understand that to those who controlled the system, medicine was first and foremost big business.

My current beliefs about the ethical correctness of practicing concierge medicine were forged on the battlefields of hospital floors,

ICUs, ERs, and in my office. My forays into local geopolitics taught me a great deal about medical ethics. These ethical lessons did not come from a textbook. They did not come from an ivory tower. They came from real life experiences as a doctor, caring for sick patients.

TUCSON, ARIZONA: GROUND ZERO FOR THE HMO MOVEMENT

When I moved to Tucson, Arizona, fifteen years ago, I knew that it was heavily penetrated by managed care. Next to St. Paul, Minnesota, there is no other place I am aware of with so many HMOs. However, I believed that I could work with the HMO executives who managed these companies. I started out trying to do so.

Shortly after going into private practice, I was struck by the number of my HMO patients who were suffering from diseases of self-abuse. Much of my large HMO panel was comprised of people who were overweight and had type 2 diabetes. Most of them did not exercise. Many had heart disease or emphysema and continued to smoke cigarettes. There was no mechanism in place to help these people make changes in their behaviors. The obvious solution to these problems was not to write more prescriptions. It was not to give people more pills. It was getting them to change their unhealthy behaviors. I knew that an ounce of prevention was literally worth a pound of cure, not only for the patient but for the HMO as well. This approach to medical care was not only shortsighted, but also expensive.

The concept of a health maintenance organization was born from the sound principle that helping people "maintain" their health could actually save the system money. It would save pain and heartache for patients as well. With healthier people, less of the healthcare dollar would have to be spent on crisis care. It made sense and was backed by scientific evidence. However, in practice, this is not how the system evolved.

A Proposal for Health Optimization

After I'd been in practice for about a year, I went to my local HMO director with a proposal. I tried to speak in her language. I said, "You understand that you are spending millions of dollars on patients who have diseases of self-abuse. They eat and drink too much. They don't exercise. They smoke. I believe that I can help you in ways that will improve your bottom line. I know that I can help your members improve their health. Many of the diseases that your members suffer from could be prevented or even 'cured' with healthier lifestyles." The director listened.

I then presented the most recent medical literature on wellness interventions. I estimated the number of cases of new type 2 diabetes the HMO could prevent by offering simple exercise programs. I talked about group nutritional counseling for diabetic members on their plan. We talked at length about *real* healthcare maintenance. She seemed genuinely interested.

I pointed out that her HMO was spending tons of money every year on useless pamphlets or other "educational materials" for its members. They had pamphlets on treating arthritis pain and headaches with an ice cube. They had pamphlets on eating vegetables. She agreed that these pamphlets contained little to no substance. This is just what they had always done.

I said, "Here is my proposal. Allow me to use the money that you are wasting on the so-called educational materials every year to develop a state-of-the-art health and fitness center in Tucson. I will design a wellness program for you and your members. I will do this free of charge, as a pilot program. It will cost you no more than you are already spending paying lip service to preventative care. If it is successful, you can use this program in other cities. It will differentiate you as "differently better" than your competition. The only way that Tucsonans will be able to join this wonderful healthcare facility will be to belong to your HMO. As opposed to your pamphlets, this will help educate and change your member's unhealthy behaviors. It will not only maintain their health but also improve it. Besides, it will save you a lot of money in the long run. What do you have to lose?"

I had the HMO director's attention. She was impressed. I was invited to the headquarters of the company in Phoenix, Arizona. Three senior executives listened to my proposal. They were polite but cool. They were more skeptical than the director in Tucson. They said that they were "interested." They told me that they would "get back to me."

A few weeks later, the director of the HMO in Tucson called me. She said, "Everyone agreed that your idea was a good one. It is progressive. It is exciting. However, those pamphlets and educational materials satisfy governmental regulations that require us to educate our patients to maintain their health. We know they are worthless, but this is a simple way to meet the governmental requirements. More to the point, we have determined that improving the long-term health of our HMO members will *not* save us any money. Our studies show that most people change their HMO plan every two to three years. If we make someone healthier over the next three years, we will only be saving money for our competition."

Such was the response from the biggest HMO in the city. The message was clear: This is about big business, doctor. It is about quarterly profits, not long-term health goals. Our short-term financial health comes before the long-term health of our members.

An HMO Report Card

As the Chairman of Internal Medicine and later as the Chief of Medicine at my hospital, I had intimate knowledge of many medical disasters that had occurred secondary to our managed care system. One of the sentinel cases was a young woman who developed a headache. The doctor had ordered an MRI of the brain. The HMO delayed granting approval. Three requests for the MRI were made by the doctor to the HMO. Each time, the doctor was mired in paperwork and phone calls. The patient's headache turned out to be due to a cerebral aneurysm. It ruptured before the MRI was ever done. The patient died. The doctor was sued. The HMO was protected under a group of laws called ERISA (Employee Retirement Income Security Act). Under the law, the HMO could not be sued for delaying care. It was the patient and the doctor who paid the price.

This disaster was only one of many stories of its kind. Stories like this adorned Tucson newspapers month after month. There was a steady stream of bad outcomes from a poorly managed, profit-based rationing of care.

In response to this problem, I formed a group called the Tucson Alliance for Medical Excellence. There were three other physician-leaders in the community who partnered with me in the group. Our mission was to study the problem of HMOs objectively; we wanted to put numbers on the complication rates. We wanted to know just how seriously medical care was being eroded in Tucson, Arizona. We decided to survey every doctor in Pima County to determine the magnitude of the problem.

I approached a statistician at the University of Arizona. Together, our group created a scientific survey designed to measure the impact of the HMOs on the quality of medical care. We paid for the survey out of our own pockets. We spent hundreds of hours on the project.

The survey was mailed to 1000 doctors. A very large number (865) of physicians responded by completing the survey. This response was in itself impressive. Doctors don't usually complete surveys. They are too busy. On January 10, 1997, the following headline ran on the front page of the *Arizona Daily Star*: "Tucson doctors say HMOs hurt medical care; 55% wouldn't enroll families in any here."

The results of the survey were as follows:

1. An overwhelming 72 percent of Tucson doctors said that HMOs hurt a doctor's ability to provide quality medical care.
2. More than 80 percent of the physicians surveyed said managed care interfered with their ability to establish good relationships with their patients.
3. As a positive, 80 percent of the physicians surveyed also said managed care had made healthcare more affordable.
4. However, when asked which of the available HMOs in the city they would select for their own families, 55 percent refused to choose, stating that *none* of the HMOs were acceptable for their own family members.

To my surprise, despite the fact that these results ran on the front page of the biggest newspaper in the city, our efforts did nothing to change the system. The three biggest HMOs did nothing to change their rationing policies. They simply ignored the article and waited for the heat to dissipate. Employers who needed to limit the financial bleeding of their businesses due to rising healthcare costs for their employees kept contracting with the HMOs.

In addition, all of the doctors who objected to the healthcare plans criticized in the survey continued to accept them. Why? Was it ethical to continue to participate in a system that was unacceptable for your own family? Physicians admitted that the HMOs damaged their relationships with their patients. They agreed that the HMOs hurt their ability to provide quality medical care. It was bad medicine! The reason they stayed was fear—fear of the financial repercussions if they dropped the managed care contracts. It was only when reimbursement dropped to 35 cents on the dollar from one of the HMOs in Tucson that many doctors resigned. This story, described as a "mutiny," was covered in *Money Magazine*.

Holding HMOs Accountable

So just how do HMOs operate? How and why do they limit care? The only way that an HMO can grow capital for its shareholders is to ration expensive care. The business model is simple. The money flowing into an HMO through Medicare and contracts with employers is fixed. Once you set rates, you can't increase those rates if the company is losing money. Profits for the company can only be maximized by limiting the flow of cash *out* of the business. If you want higher profits, tighten the screws and increase your rationing of expensive care.

Medical care delivered to HMO members consumes cash. This is why expensive tests like MRIs are frequently denied by the HMO. The HMOs hire "gatekeepers," who are specialized employees trained to ration expensive procedures and medicines. Clerical people are trained by the HMO to run through checklists to make sure that doctors on the plan are not being "capricious" with their spending. Indirectly, the doctor who participates in the plan also becomes a gatekeeper for the HMO himself. In this model, it becomes expensive for the doctor to advocate for his patients. To do so takes time. Approval for drugs and procedures requires many phone calls. Cumbersome forms must be completed. If the doctor bucks the system too frequently, he could find himself off the HMO panel all together. He could lose a significant part of his income. This is what drives the rationing behavior among doctors.

However, when you limit care and cut too many corners, people ultimately get hurt. This is what happened to the young woman with the aneurysm waiting for her MRI to be sanctioned by the HMO. Is this really just "the cost of doing business?"

Due to the number of complications and fatalities from the inappropriate rationing of healthcare in the state, the Arizona Court of Appeals decided to change the rules of the game. In 1997, the court found a way around ERISA. They discovered a way to hold the HMOs responsible for their decisions. They focused their attention on the medical doctors who held administrative positions within the HMO whose decisions were responsible for denying care. These people are called medical directors. They don't see patients any more. They ultimately make the decisions on the denial of tests like MRIs. The court ruled that medical directors, as physicians, could be held to the same level of care as a doctor at the bedside if they denied medical care as the director of a plan. As "doctors," medical directors for the HMOs were suddenly held accountable to the State Board of Medical Examiners.

As fate would have it, I was to be the first doctor in Arizona to test this new law against two local HMO medical directors. In 1998, I admitted an eighty-two-year-old patient named Jose Lopez to the hospital. Jose had been suffering from two days of intractable vomiting and chest pain. Mr. Lopez had diabetes. He had prostate cancer. He was a frail, sick man. He was not wealthy. He did not even speak English. But he was proud of the fact that he paid his insurance premium every month on time.

Eight hours after I had admitted Jose to the hospital, I was called by a nurse reviewer from the HMO. She had gone through her checklist and determined that Jose *did not meet criteria for inpatient admission.* I was told that I was wasting medical resources. Jose did not need to be in the hospital. I was told to discharge him immediately, or there would be severe consequences. I ignored the reviewer's demands. I kept Jose in the hospital.

I was called by the Lopez family a few hours later. The patient's daughter said, "Dr. Knope, my father has been vomiting for two days. He can't eat. He has diabetes. The HMO nurse just called us and said that you didn't know what you were doing. She said that our father should be discharged immediately. If he is not discharged, we will have to pay the entire hospital bill. We trust you. Please keep our father in the hospital until you discover what is wrong with him. We are poor, but we will find a way to pay for the hospitalization."

I had Mr. Lopez seen by a gastroenterologist. An endoscope was passed into his stomach. Mr. Lopez was suffering from something called severe diabetic gastroparesis. His stomach was massively dilated. It would not empty. He stayed in the hospital for two days until we could control his vomiting with medications. The HMO had egg on its face. They had no choice but to pay for the entire $9,100 of hospital bill.

I decided to test the new Arizona law. I filed a formal complaint with the State Board of Medical Examiners against the two HMO medical directors who had denied the hospitalization of Mr. Lopez. This move had huge implications. My colleagues thought I was committing professional suicide. Losing this HMO contract could have cost me my practice.

Ethics and Corruption

I was confident that I had a good case with the Board of Medical
Examiners. I was sure that they would rule in my favor. The HMO
had admitted their mistake by ultimately paying the bill. However, I
had much to learn about politics. In November of 1988, the Board
unanimously voted to dismiss my complaint. I couldn't believe it! The
story of the Board's decision again hit the front page of the paper. My
colleagues came to my defense in print.

Doctors from outside of Arizona also reacted in outrage. The story
was covered in *The Wall Street Journal*. Dr. Bernard Lown, the world-
famous Harvard cardiologist who invented the cardiac defibrillator and
later won the Nobel Peace Prize, went on the record with the *Arizona
Daily Star*. He railed against the Board's decision. He called the decision
utterly appalling. In a letter to me, he said, "This case points out that
our current medical system is no longer just incompetent, it has become
corrupt."

After I was shot down by the Board of Medical Examiners, a reporter,
Jane Erikson of the *Arizona Daily Star*, did some digging. She discovered that the lead examiner for the Board of Medical Examiners had
a serious conflict of interest. He headed a group medical practice that
had a multimillion-dollar contract with the HMO in question. It was
clear that he should have recused himself and never been part of the
investigation.

The next week, yet another front-page story ran in the *Star*, this one
exposing this conflict of interest by the Board member. Doctors from
Tucson again went on the record against the decision. However, even
after exposing the corruption, nothing changed. The HMOs claimed
that they had been vindicated by the Board. The Board claimed no
wrongdoing. The mediocrity continued.

After advocating and fighting for my patients for years in this third-
party system, I concluded that I could not change it. Neither my attempts at cooperation nor confrontation changed the system. The financial forces were too great. My meetings with HMO executives did
not work. My patient advocacy work as the Chief of Medicine did not
work. Scientific surveys documenting the magnitude of the problem
published in the newspapers did not work. State regulatory agencies
did not enforce the laws. Repeated front-page newspaper coverage did
nothing to change the way care was delivered. I finally realized that
fighting the good fight was getting me nowhere. I was not reaching my

objective of improving patient care. I was doing nothing to improve the lives of patients or doctors.

Even though the HMOs were responsible for 55 percent of my income at the time, I made a decision to drop managed care. I dropped *all* of the HMOs after the Board's decision. I went public about the fact that I could no longer practice good medicine using a fast-food model. For me, it was unethical to continue to do so.

I learned from inside sources that the HMO executives all predicted my demise. They laughed at me behind closed doors. They saw me as an idealistic, naïve young doctor. However, a very interesting thing happened after the press covered my decision to drop the plans. Every patient who was tired of HMO care in the city suddenly appeared at my door. I did not go out of business. I never even missed a payroll. My new patients were voting against a broken medical care system with their feet. I learned that there was a sizable group of people who *did* want better care and were willing to pay for it!

THE ETHICS OF CONCIERGE MEDICINE

In concierge medicine, there are no third-party payers interfering with a doctor's decision-making. The doctor is the advocate for one person only. That person is the patient. The doctor's income is not tied to the profits of the shareholders of a large company. There is no secondary financial agenda for the doctor to act as a "gatekeeper."

When I order an MRI now, there is no pressure that my medical decision is having an adverse impact 3,000 miles away on Wall Street. This has nothing to do with me or with my patient. Problems like cerebral aneurysms are handled differently in my concierge practice than they are in HMO practices. I believe that I handle them more "ethically." The case of Mitzi Thomas, noted previously, contrasts the difference.

For Harold and Mitzi Thomas, concierge medicine was a "good investment." Ethics do not even enter into the discussion. Who is being harmed by a patient paying for greater access to their doctor? Is it more ethical for doctors to handle aneurysms using an assembly-line business model where the outcome can be fatal, as opposed to a concierge medicine model where the physician is actually able to advocate for his patient?

AN IDEA WHOSE TIME HAD COME

After I left the HMOs, I learned how powerful consumer demand can be. In mid-1999, I was approached by two of my privately insured patients. They had read about this new thing called "concierge medicine." At that time, it was a novel concept. The first concierge practice had just opened in Seattle in 1996.

These patients were busy, successful businessmen. They were highly educated. They said to me, "Look, you are a smart guy. You went to an Ivy League medical school. We like your style. We like your medicine. But at best, we only have 15 minutes with you. We need more time to address our medical problems. In addition, we want you to share your knowledge about how we can stay healthy. We want greater access to you. We are willing to pay you for your services. Will you consider starting a concierge medical practice in Tucson?"

At first, I was skeptical. However, I listened to what they were saying. It made sense. One of my patients went on to say, "You are responsible for making life and death decisions on me. You look tired all the time. You see too many patients. I don't want the guy who has my life in his hands tired and worn out. I want him to be fresh. I want him to be well rested. I want him to enjoy his life and have time with his family. Are you actually fulfilled professionally by having to see so many patients?"

The need for better medical care was being driven not by ethics, not by HMOs, and not by the government. It was being driven by common sense. It was being driven by the demands of my patients for better care. There was an utter rationality to this idea that I could not ignore. However, it represented a big change. I had to reexamine all of my previously held beliefs. I had to do a lot of soul searching. I had to mentally retool.

I started my concierge program as a pilot project with just four patients. I retained my insured and Medicare patients who had been with me for years. My concierge practice soon grew to twelve patients. The idea spread by word of mouth. I was soon doing more and more concierge medicine. My patients loved it, and so did I. I had more time to practice the art of medicine after dropping the HMOs. As a result, I felt as if *all* of my patients got better care; even those on Medicare and traditional insurance.

A WARNING SHOT FROM UNCLE SAM

After I had been practicing concierge medicine for about four years, it was brought to my attention that certain politicians had concierge medicine in their sights. They didn't like it. There were some who argued that this might be a violation of Medicare guidelines. Though an investigation by the Secretary of Health and Human Services, Tommy Thompson, found no Medicare violations in the concierge model, it was becoming a political issue.

Medicare has strict rules about what a doctor can and cannot charge for his services. When I was a Medicare provider, I could only bill the discounted rate that Medicare set for me. If I were to charge a patient more than what Medicare allowed, I would be fined. I could not ask the patient to make up the difference between my rates and Medicare's rates. Furthermore, I could not even waive the co-pay for a patient who was having financial difficulty on Medicare. It was against the law. I had to charge everyone a Medicare co-pay of $6.25 for each visit.

I subsequently learned that a doctor in the Midwest who was practicing a bastardized form of concierge medicine was fined an undisclosed amount of money by Medicare. This doctor apparently sent out a letter asking all of his patients to pay an additional $400 per year for "undisclosed services," on top of accepting Medicare dollars for his visits. Though I was not doing anything like this, I learned that the Office of the Investigator General had issued a special alert to all doctors who practiced concierge medicine. Concierge physicians were instructed to consult with their attorneys to make sure that nothing they were doing was in violation of Medicare rules.

THE FINAL STEP TOWARD PRIVATIZATION

After consulting with two nationally recognized healthcare attorneys on the Medicare issue, I learned that straight answers from the government are hard to come by. When the government issues a warning of this kind, there is no one to really tell you what it means. The legal experts I consulted said that they had contacted Medicare and asked them to be specific about what did and what did not constitute a Medicare violation in a concierge model. The answers were vague. Nobody, including the lawyers, knew how to advise doctors.

Though my attorneys said that I had not done anything to run afoul of Medicare, it was clear that there was a potential for major regulation of my professional life in the future if I stayed on the plan. I could either hire high-powered attorneys to protect me, as other concierge physicians have done, or I could leave Medicare. I did the latter.

In a final move, I decided to "opt out" of Medicare altogether. I allowed my Medicare-aged patients to stay in my practice for a nominal charge of $65 per visit. For some sick patients who could not afford my $65 fee and truly needed my care, I charged them nothing. Many of my Medicare-aged patients stayed. Some decided to move on to another doctor who would only charge them $6.25 per visit. In a town in which the majority of young and middle-aged people had an HMO plan, in a retirement town in which Medicare was a gold card in most doctors' offices, I decided to drop both.

LIFE'S REAL LESSON: DON'T WASTE TIME FIGHTING. CREATE!

When people talk to me about the "ethics" of concierge medicine, when they criticize me for abandoning the system, I reflect on my efforts to change the system. I don't argue with them. All I can say is that I was personally unable to change the system. Perhaps my approaches were too idealistic. Politics has never been my forte. Perhaps I should have engaged in larger groups, like the AMA. However, as I watch the AMA attempt to reform the system, I am unimpressed with their results. It is my opinion that any wars against the HMO model become David and Goliath stories. Given my observations, I have opted to change the system by offering a positive alternative, as opposed to fighting the status quo.

SOCIALIZED MEDICINE

Some experts who criticize concierge medicine agree with me that HMOs are unethical. They suggest that the answer to our current healthcare crisis lies in a single solution: the creation of a nationalized healthcare system. In this proposed model, all people would receive the same "excellent" level of care. It sounds good on paper. However, there have been some interesting social experiments with this model in other countries that should cause us to pause and think seriously before adopting it.

For years, the Canadian national healthcare program was touted as the flagship of their political system. Since the enactment of their nationalized healthcare program, it has been illegal for Canadian doctors to offer private medical care. This has led to long lines of patients waiting for healthcare. It has led to delays in treatment, complications, and even fatalities. However, in June of 2005, the Supreme Court of Canada struck down a ban on private healthcare on the grounds that it put patients at risk. In essence, outlawing private medical care was ruled "unconstitutional" under the Quebec Charter of Rights.

The Supreme Court case was brought by Mr. George Zeliotis, a Canadian resident who waited a year to get a hip replacement. He was told that it was against the law to pay for his surgery privately. Unlike many Canadians who simply leave their country and pay for hip surgery in the United States, Mr. Zeliotis decided to stay and fight. The suit was a joint action between Mr. Zeliotis and a Montreal physician, Dr. Jacques Chaoulli.

In a four to three majority decision by the Canadian Supreme Court, the justices ruled that Quebec could not prevent people from paying for private health insurance for procedures covered under their nationalized system. In the words of the Chief Justice of the court who wrote the decision, "*Access to a waiting list is not access to healthcare* [italics mine]."

According to a *Wall Street Journal* reporter who covered this story, Mr. Zeliotis was not worried about being known as the man who helped bring down Canada's universal healthcare system. Mr. Zeliotis told *The Toronto Star*, "No way. I'm the guy saving it." Editors of the *Journal* wrote, "If the Canadian ruling can open American eyes to the limitations of government-run health care, Mr. Zeliotis's hip just might end up saving the U.S. system too."

Interestingly, the Canadian socialized medical system not only provided poor access for the rich, it also limited access for the middle class and the poor. *All* of the citizens of Canada had the same limited access to care.

WHAT ARE THE LEGITIMATE ETHICAL CONCERNS SURROUNDING CONCIERGE MEDICINE?

I'd like to switch gears for the rest of the chapter and address some of the legitimate questions that have been raised about the ethics of concierge medicine. The criticisms raise concerns that we all need to think about.

A Limited Supply of Doctors

It is argued by some "medical ethicists" that it is unethical for concierge doctors to limit the size of their practices. The argument goes like this: There is a limited supply of qualified primary care doctors in this country. If concierge medicine becomes more widespread, if doctors cut the size of their practices, it will unfairly shift the burden to other, already overworked doctors.

This is a valid concern. There aren't enough doctors in primary care. The number of graduates of American medical colleges who are choosing a career in primary care medicine is dropping. In fact, if things do not change, the American College of Physicians has predicted a total collapse of primary care medicine. The reasons for this trend are obvious. Word has gotten out to the best and the brightest of the next generation that medicine, specifically primary care medicine, is no longer the way to make a good living. It is not a very attractive proposition for a bright, young student to take out $250,000 in student loans, go to medical school for four years and then do a three-year residency, where he earns very little, just for the privilege of working for an HMO for $100,000 per year when it is all over. However, the reasons for the "primary care shortage" have nothing to do with concierge medicine. If concierge medicine fuels an exodus from an already sinking ship, people need to look at why the ship is sinking in the first place, not disparage those who choose not to drown.

If we tell young people that they have to practice fast-food medicine to be primary care doctors, the primary care shortage will only worsen. The only people who will want to work under these conditions will be foreign medical school graduates who are fleeing an even more oppressive medicine environment in another land.

Additionally, there are big holes in the ethical argument that concierge medical doctors place an unfair burden on their colleagues. It raises the question of what a physician in the United States is obligated to do with his medical degree.

Is there some unwritten, ethical code of conduct that requires a doctor to see a large number of patients? Does a doctor have to see 150 patients per week to be ethical? Is it unethical for a doctor to use his M.D. degree to become a cosmetic surgeon or dermatologist? Should some dermatologists be allowed to focus on cosmetic procedures as others treat skin cancer?

Furthermore, is it ethical for a medical ethicist to use his M.D. degree to sit around and think about medical ethics? Couldn't someone with a Ph.D. do the ethicist's job just as well? Using the ethical argument of limited supply, would it not be more ethical for the ethicist to role up his sleeves and actually start taking care of the sick people? Isn't he shifting the burden of patient care to his already overworked colleagues? And let's not forget the doctors who choose to be medical directors. They don't see patients at all. Is it ethical to use your M.D. degree to become a medical director for an HMO?

I say this tongue-in-cheek. If you want to be a medical ethicist, this is a fine way to use your M.D. degree. We need people in the medical field asking important ethical questions. I only ask these questions to point out the hypocrisy of the argument. The argument does not hold water.

What About Abandonment?

Doctors who convert to an MDVIP style of concierge model from an existing practice face the question of what to do with their patients who cannot or choose not to stay with them. If you are a doctor carrying a panel of 3,000 patients and you reduce the size of your practice to 600, requiring all who stay to sign up for the concierge plan, what are your remaining 2,400 patients to do? Obviously, they are going to need to find a new doctor. For those people who cannot afford to pay a retainer fee, or for those who choose not to, this will be a disruption in their care.

The AMA has studied the subject of concierge medicine and has decided that it is not unethical to practice in a concierge model. However, they have provided written guidelines to concierge physicians in this regard. Transferring of care to a new doctor must be handled in a sensitive and professional manner. The concierge doctor should provide information on how patients can find a new doctor.

Caring for the Indigent

Concierge medicine will not solve the problem of caring for those individuals who have no medical care at all. However, many concierge doctors donate significant amounts of their time to care for those who have no care.

In my practice, I see many patients free of charge. I have arrangements with other doctors and organizations in Tucson to refer sick indigent patients to me. I try to make the biggest contribution to my community by seeing nonroutine matters. I am a diagnostician. I deal with challenging cases. Therefore, I do not want to see indigent patients with colds and the flu. I'm not just looking for Brownie points to counter my detractors regarding the care of "poor people." I ask my colleagues to send me their diagnostic dilemmas. This is a good use of my skills. Will it solve the problem of the indigent? No, it will not. But it doesn't hurt either.

Many of the costs that limit care of the indigent could be approached by having medical and business people work together to create solutions. For example, from a business perspective, it makes no sense to have an expensive piece of diagnostic equipment like a CT scanner or MRI scanner sit unused at night. There could be significant cost savings by having these machines run late into the night, or even 24 hours per day. Those without insurance who need care could have their CT scans scheduled in the evening, saving the system money. Nurse practitioners could deal with routine problems in the night, such as earaches in a child, as opposed to having every patient seen by an ER physician.

Tort reform would go a long way toward lowering medical costs, which would provide huge savings in the medical budget to treat the indigent. The amount of money saved by physicians ordering unneeded tests in the ER to protect themselves alone would save billions of dollars. This is but a short list of ways through which money could be carved out of the system to care for those without financial means.

Advertising "Better Medicine"

The AMA has also made the point that it is important that concierge doctors do not advertise this kind of medicine as a promise for more or better diagnostic/therapeutic services. To do so would be unethical in their policy statement. In other words, it is important that a doctor does not imply that the "best medicine" is being saved for concierge patients who pay additional fees. I am particularly sensitive to this issue, since I not only take care of the very wealthy; I also take care of the very poor.

In my view, a mixed concierge practice like mine is like flying on an airplane: all people get to the same place at the same time. I take the same care in diagnostic and treatment plans with all of my patients. I have had to get creative from time to time with my poorest patients. I'll call specialists and ask for free consultations if an indigent patient cannot afford their care. But my medical thought processes and the time I devote to difficult cases are the same.

The Problem of the "Uninsured"

Concierge medicine certainly does not address the problem of the uninsured. However, when people talk about the "uninsured," they create the sense that those without insurance are also without healthcare. This is often not the case. In most cities, the uninsured get some of the most expedient and expert medical care in the world. The problem is that they don't pay for it. We do.

At St. Mary's Hospital, where I used to work, young uninsured people in their twenties and thirties will wait until 3 A.M. to come into the ER for a sore throat, a sexually transmitted disease, or pelvic pain. They do so because there is less wait at this hour. They often do not pay their bills because they have learned that they don't have to. They get ultrasounds or CT scans done STAT through the ER at all hours of the night. A radiologist must be awakened to read those STAT studies in the middle of the night for medical–legal reasons. The radiologist will never be paid for his services. The hospital, which is obligated under the law to provide "emergency" care to the uninsured, will never be paid. This leads to tremendous financial losses for the system. However, this is a social and economic problem, not a medical problem. Concierge medicine offers *no* solutions to this problem.

Each state is dealing with the uninsured problem in a different way. In the state of Massachusetts, the legislature recently approved a bill that requires all residents to purchase health insurance. If they don't have insurance, the residents of the state will face fines and legal penalties. If people cannot afford insurance, there will be subsidy programs. However, just as those who drive a car require insurance, all people in Massachusetts require health insurance. Time will tell if this strategy will effectively deal with the problem.

STRONG DOCTORS; ETHICAL DOCTORS

I am not an ethicist. I do not pretend to be able to tell another doctor what is right or wrong for him or her. The gold standard for diagnosing coronary disease is an angiogram. But I know of no gold standard for testing whether one form of medical practice is more ethical than another. There will always be a subjective component to medical ethics.

What I do know from my own observations is that most of us make better decisions when we are strong than when we are weak. Forcing doctors into a weakened position of servitude will do little to protect the long-term health interests of the country.

We could analogize the physical strength curve in Chapter 6 to the professional strength of a doctor. If he is continually challenged and has time to invest in his profession and then rest, he will get stronger. If he is "overtrained" and gets no rest, he will malfunction like an overworked athlete. If he stops investing energy in medicine due to an oppressive system, he will atrophy and become weaker over time.

My concierge practice has given me more time to become stronger as a doctor. Since I've operated a concierge practice, I've been more creative. I've developed childhood obesity programs in my community for kids with limited financial and educational resources. I've begun a relationship with physicians at the University of Arizona to soon train residents and fellows in the art of applying exercise physiology to patient care. These are creative endeavors that I believe have value to the community. I can do this because I am stronger financially and professionally. I can do this because I have time.

Most doctors go into medicine with noble aims of helping people. It gives their lives meaning. An improved system of healthcare delivery would allow them to pursue that goal creatively and come up with doctor-driven solutions to medical and societal problems rather than hampering them with overwork and paperwork.

Adopting shortsighted "ethical" positions that subjugate doctors will be counterproductive for good healthcare in the long run. Whether subjugation comes in the form of governmental regulations or financial pressures from third-party payers, the end result will be the same. What we should do instead is plan for the long run. We should explore models like concierge medicine that make the practice of medicine more rewarding; more rewarding for the patient *and* more rewarding for the doctor. In so doing, the profession will once again attract the best and the brightest in our society.

CHAPTER 9

How to Evaluate Your Current Medical Care

I'd like you to grade your current medical care on a gut level, without thinking about it for very long. Based upon your interactions with your physician to date, give your doctor an overall grade from A to E.

A   B   C   D   E

Now that you've registered your initial opinion, I'd like to refine the process by looking at several individual components of doctoring that I believe are part of overall good care. You are going to rate your doctor on his ability to address these components using the same A to E scale above. This is not an exhaustive list but the fundamental standards that should not be left out.

Staying with our principle that putting numbers on any assessment sharpens our thinking (like examining the value of your financial or health portfolios), we are going to do the same with evaluating your present medical care. After going through individual criteria, you will calculate a final grade for your doctor using the worksheet at the end of this chapter. You can see if your initial gut-level impression squares with your numerical evaluation. If you take the time to complete this exercise, it will also help you define what it is you are looking for in a physician, even if some of your criteria are a little different from mine.

Though every grading system has its limitations, we cannot escape grades. We are all evaluating each other on a regular basis, either off-the-cuff or in a more systematic way. If you are going to evaluate something as important as your medical care, you might as well put pen to paper as opposed to relying on instinct alone.

CHARACTERISTIC NUMBER ONE: HEALTHCARE ADVOCACY

In today's complicated healthcare environment, I can think of no more important role for a primary care physician than that of medical advocate. Given the complexity of modern medical science, the vast and varied options for diagnosing and treating diseases (like prostate cancer), and the very real possibility of getting fragmented medical care when you are hospitalized, you need someone who is clearly in charge of your care. This professional should also be motivated to care about what happens to you as a person.

Because of the complexity of modern diagnostics and treatments, patients often have several physicians involved in their care, not to mention physicians' assistants, nurse practitioners, and other healthcare workers. For example, if a patient has been treated for breast cancer, she may have had three separate oncologists—a surgical oncologist, a medical oncologist, and a radiation oncologist. If we presume that she also had an internist and a gynecologist at the time of her treatment, she will have had five doctors, all of whom were either prescribing drugs or delivering treatment with potential side effects and interactions.

With multiple physicians in the mix, who is the patient's ultimate medical advocate? Who is coordinating the medical care and looking out for the big picture? Are the specialists communicating with each other? If not, who makes the phone calls? Are all of the drugs she is taking compatible with one another? Does each specialist know what the other specialists are prescribing?

Treating a patient without a team leader is comparable to flying a jetliner without a captain in the cockpit. It just doesn't make sense. Ah! But I'm being overly dramatic, you say, comparing medical care to flying an airliner. Perhaps not. Hospitals are now hiring pilots and airline industry professionals to help them create systems to prevent the all-too-common medical mistakes that occur and cause a patient to crash. It may surprise you to know how few systems are in place at present to minimize medical mistakes.

In addition to advocating during times of crisis, your doctor should also be working toward the goal of fostering your optimal health. Does your doctor advocate for your wellness? Does she have a plan to get you healthier? Does she have the time to do so and follow it up? Does your doctor make sure that you are up-to-date with all of your vaccinations? Does she talk with you about exercising regularly, eating well, and maintaining a healthy body composition? Does she make sure that you are getting all of your important preventative care, such as mammograms, colonoscopies, and bone density studies?

Based upon this broad definition of a medical advocate, grade your primary care doctor regarding her ability to captain your medical team and to look out for your overall healthcare.

A   B   C   D   E

CHARACTERISTIC NUMBER TWO: TRAINING AND REPUTATION

The most important formative educational years of any physician's life occur during medical school and residency training. In this intense period, young doctors are deeply immersed in the study of medicine. They are exposed to important role models whose behavior helps shape their professional ideals. It is only natural that you would want to know from which medical school your doctor graduated. However, what conclusions you draw from this information may be of limited value.

I went to college and graduate school on the East Coast, where there was an almost neurotic attention to academic pedigree. This neurosis started with the parents and spread like a virus to their children, often beginning with the prep school a child attended and ending with his or her professional school. In medicine, the problem is that determining what defines the "best medical school" is very difficult if not impossible. Schools have different educational missions. Some schools train doctors for a career in academic medicine, while others emphasize a curriculum geared toward careers in community medicine. What may be a great school for a career in academia may not be the best school for a budding family practitioner.

Furthermore, I am aware of no study documenting any correlation between where someone went to medical school and what kind of physician they ultimately became. This is especially true in clinical medicine. This may be due to the fact that being a good doctor requires habits of lifelong learning. The medical school years are only a snapshot in time, and academic success does not guarantee long-term success as a doctor.

Though it may seem quite subjective, professional reputation is probably a far better gauge of physician quality than where the doctor trained. I know where very few of my colleagues graduated from medical school, but I can tell you in an instant whom I would call if I had a medical problem myself and whom I would never refer my patients to see.

Despite its apparent subjectivity and lack of formal criteria, it is interesting how consistent a doctor's reputation is among his or her colleagues. Being trained as careful observers, doctors are very good at sizing each other up. It is a rare case where a doctor is considered an astute clinician by some of his colleagues and a bum by others. When this happens, politics is usually at play.

Interestingly, this consistency in reputation does not always hold true when we examine a doctor's reputation among his patients. A good bedside manner can cover up a lot of medical incompetence and give the impression to the untrained that a problem doctor actually knows what he is doing. I've chaired medical committees that have been forced to take away the hospital privileges of grossly incompetent doctors. Despite documentation of their repeated complications, it is not unusual to learn that these bad apples have loyal patient followings.

The take-home message is to get, whenever possible, the opinions of physicians in your community regarding any doctor you are seeing or considering seeing. Ask specialists you know whom they recommend as an internist, family doctor, or pediatrician. If your neighbor is a reputable doctor, ask him about your doctor's reputation. Listen for pauses and look for telling body language whenever you ask about the opinion of another doctor. Even if a doctor will not tell you anything negative about a colleague, the lack of positive response can be equally important.

Finally, try finding out whom doctors see for their own primary medical care. Just ask a doctor who his doctor is. The old idea of seeing "a doctor's doctor" is not a bad policy to follow.

Circle the letter that best corresponds to your doctor's reputation in the medical community.

A   B   C   D   E

CHARACTERISTIC NUMBER THREE: BOARD CERTIFICATION

Less subjective than where someone went to medical school is whether they are board-certified in their specialty. Board certification defines a minimal level of competence established by a group of physicians within a specialty. The American Board of Internal Medicine, the American Board of Family Medicine, and the American Board of Pediatrics are three such certifying organizations.

Board certification requires the successful completion of an approved residency program in the specialty and then a rigorous written examination. In the old days, board certification never expired, and so doctors could get board-certified early in their careers and let their skills slide as they aged without losing their certification. We used to make fun of these old geezers when I was in medical school and complain that the boards should implement some standard of recertification. Medical boards finally recognized the problem and did just that, so now medical boards require ongoing assessments and recertification with periodic exams throughout a doctor's professional career. For example, to remain board-certified by the American Board of Internal Medicine, a physician must complete several open-book examinations and take an all-day exam every ten years. The process is no fun, but it helps keep doctors up-to-date.

Though board-certification is no guarantee of excellence and certainly not of good judgment, it does tell you that your doctor has completed a rather rigorous testing process overseen by a national medical organization and has also been willing to put himself through a process of unpleasant examinations to make sure that he continues to operate from a modern database of information. It tells you something about his commitment as well.

Ask your doctor or his staff if he is board-certified in his specialty. This information can also be obtained from your insurance company if your doctor takes a third-party insurance plan.

Board Certification: Yes   No

CHARACTERISTIC NUMBER FOUR: LISTENING AND CHEMISTRY

For most people, a relationship with a physician is a very personal one. Doctors, like patients, come in all flavors. Some people like a no-nonsense, factual style and need little in the way of handholding. Others prefer a more sensitive soul and a gentle approach. There is no such thing as a one-size-fits-all ideal for personality and style in a doctor. It is just a matter of personal preference and chemistry between two individuals.

Having said this, there is one personal attribute that all physicians must have if they are to be competent and effective doctors: the ability to *listen*. Ask yourself this important question: Does your doctor listen to you? Is he fully present during your visits, or does he seem distracted by the day-to-day hassles of running his practice? During visits, does he talk more about himself or his most recent vacation than he does about your health? Does he cut off your questions instead of hearing you out? Is he dismissive of your concerns before you finish explaining them?

In a recent study published in the *Annals of Internal Medicine* in June of 2007, researchers examined how often doctors talked about themselves during medical visits. After doctors agreed to participate in the study, mock patients were periodically sent into the office for medical visits which were recorded and analyzed by outside observers. Doctors in this study shared personal information with their patients during one-third of office visits. Despite the fact that many doctors believed that sharing personal information improved their ability to connect with the patient, about 85 percent of the time it was deemed unhelpful to the patient's care. Most disconcerting was the fact that once a doctor started down the road telling his own story, he rarely returned to the patient's original complaint. The study concluded that when doctors took time during the visit to personalize with a story of their own, they wasted precious time in helping their patient. Injecting the doctor's life into the visit was in fact counterproductive.

Please circle the grade that you would give to the personality match you have with your doctor. Circle a separate grade for his ability to listen.

Personality Match:	A	B	C	D	E
Grade as Listener:	A	B	C	D	E

CHARACTERISTIC NUMBER FIVE: TIME WITH AND ACCESS TO YOUR DOCTOR

To spend quality time with you, your doctor must first give you more than a few minutes per visit. Do you have adequate time with your physician, or do you feel hurried during your visits? Does your doctor ask that important final question mentioned earlier: "Is there anything else you would like to discuss today?"

What about access? If you call your doctor and ask for an appointment—say, with back pain—how long does it take to get into the office? What if you call with a potentially more serious issue, such as a fever? If your doctor is not available herself, does she have a "physician extender" such as an assistant or nurse practitioner who is able to see you? What is the quality of this person? Do you see this person more than you see your doctor?

If you leave a telephone message for your doctor, does she get back to you in a timely fashion? Is there an adequate after-hours backup system for emergencies?

Once you get into the examining room, how much time does the doctor have to spend with you? Have you ever looked at your watch and measured how much face-to-face time you share with your doctor during an average visit?

Rate your doctor in the areas of accessibility and availability.

A   B   C   D   E

CHARACTERISTIC NUMBER SIX: HOSPITAL CARE

If you've ever been hospitalized, did your doctor go to the hospital, or did he turn your care over to another doctor called a "hospitalist"? If you've never been hospitalized, now is the time to ask what would happen if you were.

As I mentioned previously, many doctors feel that they can no longer afford to go the hospital due to falling reimbursement by third-party payers and the need to stay in the office churning out patients. Especially if they are nearing the end of their careers and find it very difficult to be awakened in the middle of the night, other doctors prefer to avoid the stresses of caring for seriously ill patients.

You will have to determine how important it is for you to have your own physician care for you in the hospital when you are at your sickest. However, from my perspective, this is just when you most need your personal physician as your medical advocate—to check your medicines carefully, to look at what is hanging in the IV bags, to make sure that the best specialists are being called in on your care and to personally review all X-rays and CT scans with the radiologists.

When you go through the trouble of selecting a doctor, I hope you make a significant investment of time and energy in the process. Any physician can deal with a cold or minor scrape. The purpose of finding the right doctor is to ensure you're in good hands when you need a little more intellectual horsepower and dedication.

Find out if your doctor still maintains hospital privileges and uses them.

Yes   No

CHARACTERISTIC NUMBER SEVEN: PREVENTATIVE CARE

In addition to providing crisis care for serious medical illnesses, it is the standard of care for primary care physicians to offer healthcare maintenance advice to all patients. These kinds of services include mammograms and pap smears for women, prostate exams and PSA testing for men, vaccinations, colonoscopies, age-appropriate blood screening, and so on.

In addition, I would argue that an annual physical exam, though not advocated by all major medical organizations, is prudent. It may not seem cost-effective for Medicare to pay for everyone over the age of sixty-five in this country to have a complete annual physical, but any practicing physician will admit that he has occasionally found critically important new findings during a routine physical that resulted in an earlier diagnosis and benefit to the patient. It is often during the comprehensive visit of your annual physical exam that the doctor will take the time to make sure that you are up-to-date with all of your preventative care and to go through the chart carefully to make sure that nothing has fallen through the cracks.

How would you rate your physician in terms of providing you with an annual physical exam, encouraging you to comply with standard recommendations for preventative care, and being proactive with your healthcare maintenance?

A   B   C   D   E

CHARACTERISTIC NUMBER EIGHT: EXERCISE AND NUTRITION

If you buy my argument that there are indeed three critical components to healthcare, you will want the help of your physician in personalizing exercise and nutritional programs. I would argue that being physically active, though alone not sufficient for optimal health, is absolutely necessary to it. I would take the position that being overweight is not a matter of appearance or vanity but something that puts your most precious asset at risk. There is good evidence to say that it matters very much what you eat. So if your doctor is interested in your long-term health, these issues are worth taking the time to address.

How would you grade your physician on his knowledge and willingness to provide personalized recommendations on exercise, nutrition, and fat loss where necessary?

A   B   C   D   E

FINAL GRADE WORKSHEET

Now that you've rated your doctor in these individual areas, we are going to calculate a final grade for your current medical care as follows:
Transfer all the grades you have given above to the worksheet below.

Healthcare Advocacy:	A(4.0)	B(3.0)	C(2.0)	D(1.0)	E(0)
Professional Reputation:	A(4.0)	B(3.0)	C(2.0)	D(1.0)	E(0)
Board-Certification:	Yes(4.0)		No(2.0)		
Personality Match:	A(4.0)	B(3.0)	C(2.0)	D(1.0)	E(0)
Ability to Listen:	A(4.0)	B(3.0)	C(2.0)	D(1.0)	E(0)
Time & Access:	A(4.0)	B(3.0)	C(2.0)	D(1.0)	E(0)
Hospital Privileges:	Yes(4.0)		No(2.0)		
Preventive Care:	A(4.0)	B(3.0)	C(2.0)	D(1.0)	E(0)
Exercise & Nutrition:	A(4.0)	B(3.0)	C(2.0)	D(1.0)	E(0)

Add the total number of points: _____
Divide the total number of points by 9: _____

Find the final grade by circling the closest corresponding number to your final calculation.

$$4.0 = A$$
$$3.5 = B+$$
$$3.0 = B$$
$$2.5 = C+$$
$$2.0 = C$$
$$1.5 = D+$$
$$1.0 = D$$
$$0.5 = D-$$
$$0.0 = F$$

What you do with this final grade will be up to you. If you are happy with your overall medical care, you have learned something very important. If there are only one or two areas where you feel your medical care falls short, perhaps you could ask your doctor to try to meet your needs. If you gave your doctor a final grade of D+, you may want to find someone more qualified to protect and manage your health assets.

CHAPTER 10

Making Your Concierge Medicine Investment Affordable

So, you've made the decision to invest in your health. You agree that your health is your most precious asset. You buy into the idea that concierge medicine has real value. However, you also live in the real world with a real world budget. You don't have unlimited investment capital, like those people who have joined the MD^2 practice in Seattle.

This chapter is written for those people who cannot simply write a check for the concierge medicine program of their choice without thinking about it. I will assume that the reader of this chapter is interested in a concierge program that costs between $1,600 and $5,000 per year. I will assume that the reader of this chapter would like to make concierge medicine as cost-effective as possible.

Unlike the other chapters in this book, I am going to suggest that you read this chapter selectively. Use it as a reference chapter depending on your financial situation, your age, your health, and your interest in learning about insurance options.

HOW TO USE THIS CHAPTER

1. If you have the capital to invest in the concierge program of your choice, I suggest that you skip this chapter.
2. If you can afford a concierge plan by simply trimming a little fat from your budget in other areas (maybe cigarettes, designer coffee, or your

200 channel cable TV bill) you may want to skip this chapter as well. As I've stated earlier, MDVIP offers concierge care for the price of a pack of cigarettes per day.

3. However, if you or your family members are relatively healthy but have a limited amount of capital to invest in a concierge program, you should read this chapter carefully, particularly the section about a new insurance option that might well allow you to purchase concierge care for the same or even less than you are presently paying for your healthcare. You may want to consider purchasing something called a health savings account (HSA) coupled with a high-deductible health plan.

4. If you are of Medicare age and are looking for ways to make concierge medicine affordable, you will not be eligible to purchase an HSA and may want to skip these pages. However, you may be able to afford concierge care by taking advantage of the new savings that have been created by the government in the form of Medicare Part D, which helps with the cost of drugs. I will discuss this subject briefly later in this chapter.

5. Finally, if you are chronically ill and cannot get inexpensive health insurance, you are going to need some professional help. I will discuss this problem as well.

A LEGITIMATE DISCLAIMER

Because I am *not* a health insurance specialist, an accountant, or a lawyer, I will give you a general warning before you read this chapter. This chapter is *not* a substitute for a consultation with your professionals in your own state. Because insurance laws vary from state to state, and because everyone's health insurance needs are unique, you will need to consult with your own experts before following any of the options that I have put forth in this chapter. If you are considering finding a doctor through a group like MDVIP (www.mdvip.com), you may want to consult them regarding laws in your state. The Society for Innovative Medical Practice Design, SIMPD (www.simpd.org), is an additional reference. Finally, when you interview potential concierge doctors, ask them how the laws of your state work in regards to concierge medicine.

Use this chapter as a way to boost your general knowledge on health insurance, to become more aware of the new healthcare options, and to approach your experts with intelligent questions.

SECTION I: OPTIONS FOR YOUNG AND MIDDLE-AGED HEALTHY PEOPLE

I am going to begin this chapter by exploring ways for young to middle-aged, relatively healthy people to make concierge medicine affordable. If you are in this group and are presently insured through a plan offered by your employer or though a group plan, read on.

The New Laws of 2004

In 2004, the Bush administration enacted some exciting and revolutionary new laws that give you, the consumer, greater choices and freedom to purchase affordable health insurance. Chances are you don't know much about these new laws. Most people don't. The government has not done a very good job of educating the public. Unfortunately, health insurance is a complex subject. It can't be explained in an easy-to-read pamphlet. Furthermore, these laws were tainted with partisan politics. Regardless of your political persuasion, these laws offer many Americans health insurance options that they did not have in the past.

The idea behind the new laws was to entice individuals to take financial responsibility for their own health insurance as opposed to relying on the government or employers to pay for their healthcare expenses. Both government and big businesses have a lot to gain if people start paying for more of their own healthcare insurance. The enticement for you to engage in such behavior comes in the form of some considerable tax breaks and a great deal more freedom in your healthcare choices.

The government has made it attractive for individuals to purchase their own high-deductible health insurance plans linked to an HSA. What this means is that for a relatively small amount of money, you or your family can purchase catastrophic health insurance for a minimal monthly premium. This premium is much lower than that of a traditional health insurance plan, typically about half the cost. In addition, you can save some of the money that you would have normally paid your employer for traditional health insurance in a special savings account for your future healthcare needs. This is the "health savings account" component of the program.

Note that this new kind of health insurance is purchased by you as an individual. Your employer does not buy it for you. It is yours to keep. It is not subject to changes in your employment. You can't lose it if you lose your job. It follows you if you change jobs. Even if you own and operate your own small business, you keep your individual health insurance even if you sell or lose your business due to disability, bankruptcy, or any other changes that might occur in your life. In this way, it is more secure than a plan that is dependent on your present employer.

What Are the Benefits of the New Insurance Laws?

One of the biggest benefits of these new plans is that they allow you to purchase healthcare with *pretax dollars*. However, the benefits go beyond this. The new laws of 2004 offer you the following additional advantages:

- Catastrophic healthcare coverage at an affordable price.
- Greater options to choose your own doctor and specialists.
- Tax incentives to put away money for your future healthcare needs.
- Tax breaks in paying for wellness care, medically prescribed weight loss programs, medications and even over-the-counter medications.
- Tax breaks to pay for additional health services such as dental care and vision care, which are often not part of traditional insurance plans.

Just What Is a Health Savings Account?

A health savings account is an interest-bearing savings account that allows you to put away tax-free money for your future healthcare needs. At the present time, an individual may put up to $237.50 per month in pretax dollars into their own private HSA. A family may put up to $470.83 per month in pretax dollars into their HSA. So in the calendar year of 2007, a single person might have saved up to $2,850 and a family might have save up to $5,650 for future medical costs. Each month that this money is not used for medical care, it continues to grow with interest. It is important to know that each year the government sets new limits on how much you can contribute to your HSA. For example, in 2008, an individual will be able to contribute $2,900 per year and a family $5,800 per year.

If you need money to pay for immediate healthcare expenses, such as a doctor's visit, you simply write a check from your HSA. If you go to your dentist, you can pay for the visit with pretax dollars, using your HSA. If you need to pay for drugs, you can do so with your HSA. If you need new eyeglasses, use your HSA.

If you do not have any medical expenses during the year, the money in your HSA simply rolls over into the next year. It continues to gain compound interest and grows until you do need it. Each year, the amount that you can contribute increases slightly and is set by the U.S. government.

Over time, you can save a lot of tax-free money for future medical care. At the age of sixty-five, you can no longer contribute to your HSA. However, everything that you have put into the account is yours for your lifelong medical expenses.

The Benefits of an HSA

The tax-deductible benefits of an HSA are numerous:

- First, your taxable income is reduced by opening an HSA. This is because the money that you pay into your HSA is deducted from your income before you pay your taxes.
- Second, you do not pay taxes when you take money out of your HSA for medical expenses. (This is different than a 401K plan, where you invest with pretax dollars but must pay taxes on any earned income when you take that money out after retirement.)
- Third, you pay *no* taxes when you spend HSA money to pay for doctors' visits or any other legitimate medical expense.

From a tax perspective, the HSA is a triple whammy in your favor. You reduce your taxable income. You pay no taxes on the money that you save for healthcare. You pay no taxes when you take the money out of the account. In addition, you pay no taxes when you purchase your healthcare.

Contrast an HSA with a typical health plan. If you pay the doctor or the dentist for a traditional office visit, you are paying his or her bill with after-tax dollars. If you are in a 30 percent tax bracket, you only keep $70 of every $100 that you earn in salary after taxes. To generate $100 in after tax income to pay that $100 office visit, you have to earn $142. Therefore, the real cost of a $100 doctor's visit is $142 in pretax dollars.

What Is a High-Deductible Health Insurance Plan?

To be eligible to open an HSA, you must first purchase a high-deductible insurance plan. You cannot open an HSA without such a plan. The two are linked. High-deductible health plans are now offered by many large insurance companies such as Blue Cross Blue Shield, Aetna, and United Healthcare.

The purpose of a high-deductible health insurance plan is to lower your monthly insurance costs in exchange for the company covering only those expensive, catastrophic medical problems that most healthy people rarely have. A high-deductible plan does not pay for routine healthcare costs. It covers serious medical problems only—those problems that would otherwise drive you into bankruptcy, such as an accident, an unforeseen hospitalization, a surgery, or an obstetrical catastrophe.

In purchasing a high-deductible insurance plan, you have many options regarding how much you want your annual deductible to be. Your deductible can be as low as $1,000 per year for your healthcare costs. This means that you would pay the first $1,000 in medical expenses before the plan kicks in. Alternatively, you can purchase a plan with a deductible as high as $5,650 per year for a family. This means that you would be responsible for the first $5,650 in medical expenses every year, provided that you needed to spend anywhere near this much money (which is uncommon for many healthy families). However, even in a bad year, you would pay for those first $5,650 in expenses using tax-free dollars from your HSA. In contrast to high-deductible plans, most people who have a traditional health insurance plan have a low deductible of around $500 for the year.

Because most people are relatively healthy, they usually do not benefit from the extra expense of a traditional, low-deductible health plan. Many healthy people don't even reach their $500 deductible each year. This is because they don't have large health expenditures in most years. The average person sees his or her doctor only a few times during a twelve-month period. The downside of a low-deductible plan for a relatively healthy person is that it is very expensive.

The irony of low-deductible health plans is that many people are already paying for most, if not all, of their doctors' visits without realizing it, on top of paying through the nose for catastrophic coverage. Consider a typical scenario. If you see the doctor five times in a year, at $100 per visit, you will just meet your $500 deductible by the end of that year. At the end of the year, you will have paid for all of those five doctor visits on your own. In addition, you will have paid for those doctor visits using after-tax dollars. If you used after-tax dollars to pay for those visits (in a 30 percent tax bracket), you would have actually spent $714 in pretax dollars for those five visits. In addition, you would have paid an expensive monthly premium, based upon the fact that you had a low deductible.

This approach does not make sense for many people. *The primary value of insurance is to prevent personal bankruptcy should you have a serious medical problem.* What most people are effectively doing on a traditional insurance program (unbeknownst to them) is *prepaying* their medical care. I'll explain this fact later on in the chapter.

By contrast, in a high-deductible plan, you pay insurance premiums to cover only the very expensive, unforeseen medical disasters you might encounter. This is what insurance was originally designed to do. With a high-deductible plan, it is now possible for the average thirty-year-old male to obtain catastrophic health insurance for around $100 per month. The average single female can obtain the same coverage for around $125 per month. The savings to the average healthy person by switching from a low-deductible to a high-deductible strategy can be huge. The amount of money saved by increasing your deductible can then be used to invest in individualized healthcare, such as a concierge medical plan if you so desire. This has the potential to increase the quality of care and broaden your choices.

The Benefits of Having Your Own Insurance Plan

Even if you own your own business and have lots of money, consider this: If you get your health insurance through a group plan in your business, your health insurance is tied to your business. If you later become sick or disabled and close your business, you will lose your insurance plan. Now, if this occurs, you will have to find individual healthcare insurance with a new serious medical condition. Good luck! Many companies will not insure someone with a serious medical problem. If they do, it will cost you an arm and a leg in premiums. In this regard, it may be wise even for wealthy small business owners to purchase their own individual health insurance using the strategy above. This is precisely what I have done for myself and my family. I dropped my low-deductible plan and purchased a high-deductible health plan with an HSA. Even if I leave my medical practice, our health insurance will remain intact.

How Insurance Works

Before we start looking at how much money you might save using a high-deductible/HSA strategy, we have to define what insurance is and how it works. In the simplest terms, insurance is a promise of reimbursement for a large, unexpected expense. It is an agreement between you and your insurance company that says you will be financially compensated in the event of some unforeseen catastrophic financial loss.

Property insurance, for example, is designed to protect the financial consequences of the loss of your stuff. As a person with material assets, you pay monthly premiums for any potential losses that you might suffer by entering a risk pool with other people who also pay monthly premiums to protect their stuff. Since everyone in that risk pool will not have a simultaneous property loss, the insurance company is able to pay you when lightning strikes your home or property. The company also collects enough in premiums from each member so that there is plenty of cash left over in the till, which provides a hefty profit for the CEO and the Wall Street investors.

Similarly, the purpose of health insurance is to prevent personal bankruptcy should you suffer a costly medical illness. Financial devastation can occur with any serious medical problem. Hospital bills and the cost of cancer drugs can put you in the poorhouse by themselves. A diagnosis such as cancer and heart disease or a car accident can send almost anyone into personal bankruptcy.

However, in our culture, the term "health insurance" has been distorted. It has come to mean much more than catastrophic financial coverage for unforeseen health disasters. Health insurance has evolved differently than property insurance. For many people, health insurance means having their *entire* healthcare bill paid for in one "convenient" monthly premium, with a significant portion of this bill paid by employers. The premium is marketed to cover doctors' visits, blood tests, diagnostic procedures, hospitalizations, and all other medical needs, with the promise that you will only pay an out-of-pocket $500 in any given year, no matter what happens to you.

The problem with this method of paying for health "insurance" is that it is a very expensive way to purchase "healthcare." Technically speaking, this is *not* insurance at all.

Health Insurance vs. Property Insurance

To illustrate the problems with traditional health insurance, let me draw a contrast between health insurance and property insurance. Jim and Sally are a typical hard-working couple in their mid-thirties. They and their kids make a family of four. Their two children are healthy. No one in the family has any serious medical problems.

Jim and Sally decide to buy a new home for $250,000. The annual cost of their homeowner's insurance is pretty low at $650 per year. This is because most homes do not burn down or get hit by lightning. Jim and Sally need catastrophic insurance for their new home, just in case something bad happens.

One day their insurance agent tells Jim and Sally that they can purchase a new, super-duper form of homeowner's insurance which is analogous to health insurance. This insurance will cover them for *any and all unforeseen problems* with the home. The homeowner's plan reimburses them not only for large losses like fire; it pays for small expenses as well. Sounds good, right? If the paint on their home flakes, the "insurance plan" will pay for repainting. If little Johnny runs his bike into the garage door, the insurance company will pay. The deductible for this comprehensive homeowner's plan is very low: only $100 per year. However, the cost in annual premiums is $5,000 per year!

Jim and Sally do some research. They sit down and put a pencil to paper. They learn that the average annual cost of home maintenance and repairs is only about 1 percent of the cost of the home. In their case, with a home that costs $250,000, they should expect to pay only $2,500 per year for routine repairs. Unless there is some unlikely set of circumstances, Jim and Sally would save about $2,500 per year by paying for routine home maintenance themselves, as opposed to paying the $5,000 in annual premiums on the super-duper homeowner's plan.

Do Jim and Sally take the all-inclusive homeowner's plan at $5,000 per year? Are they seduced by the "all-inclusive benefit" of the plan? Of course not. It would be unwise to do so. You can't even buy such a comprehensive homeowner's plan. You can't buy this kind of insurance coverage for your car either. If property insurance were de-signed to cover any and all maintenance issues on your property, it would be ridiculously expensive. No one would do it. This would be tantamount to prepaying maintenance on your stuff at an exorbitant rate. However, this is precisely what Jim and Sally do with their health insurance.

Jim and Sally don't use the same critical thinking when purchasing their health insurance as they do with their stuff. The subject of health insurance confuses them, like it confuses most of us. They just pay a monthly healthcare premium to a PPO through Jim's employer for their family at a cost of about $5,400 per year. They are duped into this policy by being told that they have a low deductible of only $500 per year.

What is this low-deductible health plan really costing Jim and Sally? Jim's employer charges him about $450 per month to include his family on the plan. Jim could easily shop on the Internet and get a high-deductible health plan for his family at about half that cost. He could open an HSA and save even more money for future healthcare by saving pretax dollars. However, he doesn't understand the rules of the game. The rules are new and confusing. He "doesn't have time" to investigate them.

Until they reach their $500 deductible each year, Jim and Sally already pay the cost of their doctors' visits. They do so using after-tax dollars. Year after year, they pay $5,400 per year for this low-deductible plan, even though they don't use much in the way of medical services. The insurance company and its shareholders get rich from the ignorance.

The High-Deductible Option

What would happen if Jim and Sally were to insure their health the way that they insured their home? What if they simply went to a higher-deductible health plan? What if they paid for routine medical care out of their own pocket using pretax dollars using an HSA?

If they raised their deductible from $500 to $2,000 per year, their monthly premium would drop from $450 per month to around $200 per month. This would result in an annual savings of $3,000 for the family! Since Jim and Sally are healthy, as are about 80 percent of Americans their age, this would make a lot of sense.

Using Your Health Savings to Individualize Medical Care

Now, if Jim and Sally valued their health as the asset that it is, they could find better ways to spend that $3,000 every year on optimizing their health. They might use this money to invest in a relationship with a concierge doctor.

With $3,000 saved in health investment capital every year, they could find a doctor who has more time for them. They could invest their money in their long-term wellness. They could find a doctor to counsel them on individualizing an exercise and nutritional plan. If they were overweight, they could find a doctor who had the time to help them with weight loss. They could invest some of their money in valuable preventive care, which would pay dividends over a lifetime.

For the same cost that they are now paying for Jim's employer-based healthcare, they could get more attentive and personalized medical care. In Jim and Sally's case, the new health insurance laws could free up the money they might use to protect their most precious asset by investing in a concierge medical program. The new laws of 2004 go together with the individualized approach of concierge medicine like hand and glove.

Low-Deductible Misconceptions

Are doctor's visits really paid for on most low-deductible plans? No they are not. Not unless you see the doctor frequently every year. Even if you see the doctor every three to four months, you probably don't stop to think that you are paying out of your pocket for your doctor's visits already.

If Jim, Sally, and their two kids were to see the doctor five times over the next year at $100 per visit, they would pay out-of-pocket $500 on their traditional plan for these visits. They would pay this money directly to the physician, using after-tax dollars.

In addition, they would have to pay the $5,400 in annual premiums to their insurance company in case one of them experienced a medical disaster. This means that the true cost of their healthcare (visits plus premiums) would run almost $6,000 per year. This is a lot to pay for catastrophic medical coverage.

Viewed from a different angle, if you don't use your catastrophic coverage, this is a lot of money to pay for five brief doctor's visits. If their average doctor's visit lasts about 10 minutes, and the family had no hospitalizations over the year (which is typical), they will have spent $6,000 for about 60 minutes of face-to-face time with their physician. In effect, they will have paid about $100 per minute with the doctor or $1,000 per visit. This is rather expensive, especially when you consider this time is usually spent with an overburdened doctor who sees thirty patients per day and has no time to help you investigate a problem in depth, much less examine your long-term health goals. It is certainly not a good return on your financial investment.

During most years, this family is *prepaying* a lot of money for medical services that they will never use! They are getting no preventative care to speak of. This is not a good use of precious capital. It is not a good investment in your health.

In a typical third-party insurance plan offered by an employer, it is true that the thinking is taken out of the process for you. But for many people, the insurance company is performing a wallet biopsy in the process. Ignorance about health insurance is very costly. This is your hard-earned money; use it wisely!

Equal in importance to this waste of capital is the fact that *many prepackaged insurance plans often take away your freedom of choice regarding what doctors you can see.* They limit the hospitals that you can use. You can't always go wherever you want for your medical care in an employer-based insurance plan, especially if it involves an HMO. What if you need a consultant at the Mayo Clinic for a rare disease and your plan doesn't contract with Mayo? If you want this kind of care, you will have to pay for it out of your own pocket, using after-tax dollars. On the other hand, if you have a high-deductible HSA plan, you can take your own tax-free money and go where you want for your care. If you've saved $10,000 in your HSA and you want to use your health savings at the Mayo Clinic or a hospital in Switzerland, it is your choice.

In an MDVIP style of concierge medicine practice, the average concierge fee runs between $1,500 and $1,800 per year. Jim and Sally could take the $3,000 they would save in monthly premiums by purchasing a high-deductible plan and put this toward concierge care. With this single change in their insurance deductible and no further alterations in their budget, concierge medicine would suddenly become an affordable option. Instead of prepaying for care that they may never receive, they could have a concierge doctor who spends time with them on optimizing their health, as well as being available for crisis care.

What Are the Additional Benefits of the HSA to Jim and Sally?

If Jim and Sally purchased a high-deductible health plan, they could open that HSA. They could invest $2000 per year in tax-free dollars for their future healthcare needs, which is the amount of their annual deductible.

Here's how an HSA works. If your deductible is $1,000 per year, you can put up to $1,000 in pretax dollars in your HSA over the course of that year. If your deductible is $2,000, you can put away $2,000. Again, the maximal amount that you could have put into a tax-free HSA in 2007 was $2,850 for an individual and $5,650 for a family. This adds up every year, especially since the money grows interest. If Jim and Sally saved $2,000 every year in their HSA over the next twenty years at 4 percent interest, they would have over $66,000 to use for healthcare expenses. Just remember; you can only open an HSA if it is linked to a high-deductible health plan.

What this shows is that the HSA can become an *investment tool* for future healthcare expenses. If you start your HSA at age thirty-five and save $5,000 per year, you can roll this money over for later healthcare expenses, even for care after the age of sixty-five. All of the time that you have money in your HSA, it is gaining compound interest. If you need to pay for medical care in the interim, you simply write a check out of your HSA. Some HSAs even offer a convenient debit card to use for your healthcare expenses.

Should you become unemployed, you can still use your HSA to pay for your monthly health insurance premiums until you find another job. The HSA is very versatile. It is worth your time to become familiar with this option.

Employer-Based High-Deductible HSA Options

Because employers are trying to cut healthcare costs, many businesses are examining options to offer employer-based high-deductible HSA plans to their employees in the future. This may add another option for you as opposed to opening an individual high-deductible plan on your own. Again, consult with your accountant, doctor, and attorney when you are making these important insurance decisions.

Can You Use HSA Money to Pay for Concierge Medical Care?

The simple answer to this question is yes. Though I am not a tax expert, I can read the English language. I can read the IRS Web site, which was designed for non-accountants like me to read. According to the IRS, HSA money can be used to pay for any legitimate medical expense. I can think of no reasonable argument that could be made that the medical services offered by a concierge physician are anything but legitimate medical expenses, especially when the law allows you to pay for healthcare expenses like eyeglasses, dental care, and over-the-counter medications using HSA funds. When the question is asked regarding *who* determines what constitutes a legitimate medical expense, the IRS guidelines are clear. It is you, the HSA holder, who makes the determination regarding legitimate medical expenses, presumably after consulting with your accountant. Certainly, if you decide to use your HSA money to pay for concierge fees, consult your accountant first. Have adequate documentation of what you do. This is what I have done and what I advise my patients to do. Have your accountant review your concierge contract.

If you are able to use pretax dollars to pay for part or all of your concierge care, you will save even more money than you will save by switching from a low-deductible to a high-deductible health plan. For all of the general information that you may need regarding the kinds of medical services that can be paid for with an HSA, simply go to www.treasury.gov/offices/public-affairs/hsa/.

Comparison of a High-Deductible Plan for a Single Man or Woman

The following comparison data was prepared by a local health insurance agency in Tucson to provide some examples of how much individuals as well as a family of four might save by moving from a low-deductible to a high-deductible plan in my city. Though rates may vary from state to state, this will give you some idea about what may be possible in your hometown. As you can see, the monthly savings are significant on a high-deductible plan compared to an employer-based plan. In this analysis, monthly high-deductible payments were one-third to one-half that of traditional plans.

	Single Male (30)	Single Female (30)	Family of 4 (Male, 40; spouse, 40; and 2 children)
Typical Employer Plan $500 deductible, 80% coinsurance, $20 office visit co-pay	$300	$300	$950
Individual HSA Qualified PPO $2,600 deductible, all costs to deductible, then 100% coinsurance	$88	$125	n/a
Family (of 4) HSA Qualified PPO $5,150 deductible, all costs to deductible, then 100% coinsurance	n/a	n/a	$473

Note: Typical employer rates are an average of ten medium-sized employers in the Tucson marketplace.

The above premium numbers do not take into account the actual cost and exposure that the covered employees and family members will be exposed to. Premium costs illustrated in the example above do not take into account any employer contributions toward premiums. In the random sample of medium market employer groups, we have an average employer contribution of 70 percent toward a single employee's monthly premium and 10 percent toward dependents in the family example. In the next example you will find a more realistic representation of actual costs when an employee chooses to leave their employer-sponsored plan and secure an HSA qualified plan independently of their employer.

Family of 4 (Male, 40; spouse, 40; and 2 children)	Typical Employer Plan	Independent HSA Family Plan
Total monthly premium	$950	$473
Monthly employer contribution (70% to single employee; 0% dependents)	$210	n/a
Actual premium to employee	$740	$473
Deductible	$1,500 total family	$5,150 total family
Maximum payable under coinsurance	$3,000	n/a; coinsurance 100%
Maximum exposure (Deductible + Maximum under coinsurance)	$4,500	$5,150
Worst-case scenario (Maximum exposure + Annual premiums)	$13,380	$10,826

How Do You Open a High-Deductible Plan with an HSA?

The easiest way to begin shopping for a high-deductible plan linked to an HSA is to search the Web sites of established insurance companies. Just search for "HSA and high-deductible plans" in your favorite Internet search engine. You will see Web sites from many major insurance carriers advertising these plans. Look at prices. Shop around. Once you understand the basics, call an insurance agent and ask him to explain the plans that he carries. Then speak with your accountant before making the move.

Many banks are now offering HSAs which can be purchased separately from the health insurance company offering the high-deductible plans. If you want to put a custom program together, you can buy your insurance plan from an insurance company and select your HSA from another company or bank.

SECTION II: MAKING CONCIERGE MEDICINE MORE AFFORDABLE AFTER THE AGE OF SIXTY-FIVE

What If You Are Sixty-five or Over?

If you are sixty-five years of age or older, you will *not* be able to open an HSA under current law. However, you already have catastrophic medical care under Medicare Part A, which is a huge benefit. All of the money that you have contributed to Medicare over your lifetime is now available to you as a safety net for any unforeseen medical disasters.

If you are sixty-five or older and opt for an MDVIP-style concierge practice, your physician will bill Medicare in addition to charging you an annual retainer fee. All Medicare rules will apply to the cost of your doctor's visits. Any practice that you join will be able to explain the details of medical billing under this kind of arrangement.

Though you can't open an HSA after age sixty-five, there are other new laws that have created real savings in your medical budget and freed up potential healthcare dollars for use elsewhere. Medicare now pays for prescription drugs in the form of Medicare Part D. This benefit is available to all persons with Medicare, *regardless of income*.

Medicare helps you pay for drugs up to a limit of $2,250 in total each year. Once your total drug costs for the year reach $3,600, Medicare pays 95 percent of the costs and you pay only 5 percent for the rest of the year. For more information on the new Medicare drug benefits, go to the Medicare Web site at www.Medicare.gov.

Sadly, many seniors have not yet signed up for the Medicare Part D benefit. Just like the new insurance laws, the new drug plans are confusing. Don't let the new rules intimidate you. Find someone to help you with the new Medicare drug plan. Call your local senior citizens organization and ask how to negotiate the waters.

If you were to save several thousand dollars per year in your prescription drug costs using Medicare Part D, you would have the money available for more individualized healthcare. With this new benefit, many seniors will have more disposable income for other healthcare expenses.

SECTION III: WHAT IF YOU HAVE CHRONIC MEDICAL PROBLEMS?

HSAs work well provided that you do not have serious medical problems to begin with and are under the age of sixty-five. However, if you have a chronic medical problem and are under the age of sixty-five, it may *not* make sense for you to purchase an individual high-deductible plan. You may not even be able to find an insurance carrier willing to cover you if you have a complicated preexisting condition. You may not be able to afford a high-deductible plan if your annual medical expenses are large every year. If you already have health insurance in the setting of a serious medical condition, you would be well advised to keep your present plan and investigate what special programs might be available in your state to help you reduce your medical expenses. Again, in this situation, consult with your experts.

If one or more family members have serious medical problems, you may consider getting high-deductible insurance for the healthy family members before they develop problems. You may want to work out a separate option for the family member(s) with the difficult problems. You may need to explore options in your state that subsidize catastrophic care for people with serious preexisting problems. For an excellent reference on this subject, you may want to consult Paul Zane Pilzer's new book, *The New Health Insurance Solution*, which is also an excellent reference on HSAs and high-deductible plans.

PRIORITIZING, PLANNING, AND BUDGETING: KEEPING HEALTH COSTS IN PERSPECTIVE

So what is your health really worth to you? If you live in the average home in this country, which now costs $280,000, you are paying about $2,800 every year just to keep your home in good repair. The average car owner pays about $8,000 per year for the privilege of driving. Even if you own your own car, you still pay about $4,000 per year for fuel, upkeep, and maintenance of your vehicle. In short, most of us have no problem working hard to pay to maintain our material possessions. And it's all just stuff!

People spend thousands of dollars each year on dining out, cigarettes, alcohol, travel, and entertainment. We pay for expensive cable TV services and satellite dishes with dozens of channels. Americans now spend $8 billion per year on bottled water alone. Is it really accurate to say that you *can't* adjust your budget and come up with $1,600 per year for more effective healthcare to protect your most precious asset?

There is a lot of fat in most of our budgets. Most of us can find ways to pay for what is really important in our lives. In most cases, it is simply a matter of juggling a few expenses to come up with the needed capital to invest in what we really want in life.

Don't be like the group of wealthy businessmen that I described earlier in the book. Don't accumulate lots of wealth and lots of stuff and ignore your health. Learn the lessons that I've learned from *rich guys with heart disease*. Invest in your health. Look at your health as a long-term investment.

Talk with your local experts to see how you might make concierge medicine affordable. Visit the U.S. Department of Treasury Web site and learn about HSAs. The Web site is laid out in a simple and understandable format. If you are a senior, learn about Medicare Part D. With all of the negative news about the problems with rising healthcare costs, most people have missed the good news about President Bush's new healthcare programs in 2004. These new laws have given millions of Americans the freedom to use their own money to purchase the kind of healthcare that they deserve, but at the moment, most people are simply unaware that these options exist.

CHAPTER 11

How to Find the Right Concierge Physician for You

Okay, so you've decided that concierge medicine is for you. The question now becomes how to find the right concierge doctor.

Doctors are as diverse as any other group of professionals. Doctors have different levels of training and experience. They have different personalities. They have different specialties and areas of professional interest. Bedside manner can be as unique and interesting as the individual physician.

Signing up for a concierge program is a significant decision. Optimizing your health is a long-term commitment. You will want to find a physician who embodies those qualities that are most important to you. You will want to find a physician who views health as an asset, something to protect and grow, something that requires a proactive approach.

When you are looking for the right concierge doctor for you, you are searching for two primary qualities: *competence* and *chemistry* with the doctor.

BASIC RESOURCES

Since concierge medicine is relatively new, you may need to do some looking in your community to find a concierge doctor. You can start by looking at Web sites, like that of the Society for Innovative Practice Design (www.simpd.org). This was the first professional group of concierge doctors to formally organize. As I said earlier, this organization was originally called the American Society of Concierge Physicians.

The largest franchised group of concierge doctors, MDVIP, also has a Web site on which you can search for a concierge physician. According to *Fortune* magazine, one out of every four doctors in concierge practices is affiliated with MDVIP. Obviously, this will not be a good source if you are interested in one of the other two concierge medicine models, such as the MD^2 model or a mixed practice model like mine.

Many concierge physicians have their own Web sites. You can search the Internet by putting in terms like "concierge medicine" or "retainer medicine" and linking the term to the name of your city. You may also want to contact your county medical society for the names of doctors who provide concierge medicine services. Local hospitals also have physician referral services that may be able to point you in the right direction.

INTERVIEWING A CONCIERGE DOCTOR

Once you have found the name of a concierge doctor, you will want to call and ask about the program. If the practice sounds appealing to you over the phone, you will want to arrange an interview. The interview is the most important part of the selection process.

Interviewing policies differ from doctor to doctor. If the concierge doctor does not offer an interview, consider looking for another doctor. You do not want to enter into an arranged medical marriage without ever having met your healthcare partner. If the doctor's position is that he is too busy to sit down and talk with you about his program, find someone else.

I offer a complimentary 30-minute consultation to anyone interested in my practice. This is a chance for prospective patients to get to know me. It is also an opportunity for me to get to know them. If I don't think I can meet someone's needs, I will be honest with them.

To get the most out of the experience, you will need to approach the interview with a plan. Like any other interview, meeting with a doctor is *not* just a cordial conversation. Of course you want the meeting to be pleasant. After all, you are hoping that this person will become your doctor for years to come. However, unlike a free-flowing conversation between friends, you should have an *agenda* for this meeting. You are interviewing this professional to acquire information to make an informed decision about whether or not he is the right person to manage your health assets. I'm not advising you to walk in like a skeptical consumer shopping for a new car. Don't be defensive. Just go into the interview with some questions in mind.

What Questions to Ask

The first priority in interviewing a doctor is to find out who he really is. What is his training? What is his background and experience? What kind of person is he? Is he an internist or family practitioner? An internist is a specialist in adult medicine, whereas a family practitioner usually cares for children as well. A family practitioner may also offer obstetrical and gynecological care.

The best way to start the interview is by asking the doctor *open-ended questions*. Let the doctor talk. Let him tell you who he is and what his practice is all about. I start my interviews by asking the patient if *they* would like to begin with their questions or if they would like me to give them an overview of my practice. I do this out of courtesy. It is the patient's interview. However, to get the most out of your interview, I would advise you to ask the doctor to speak first. In this way, you will learn much more about *him*.

What I mean by asking open-ended questions is to start out by being very general. Say something like, "Could you please tell me what your practice is all about?" or "How does your concierge medicine practice work?" This will give you a chance to see how the doctor expresses himself. It will tell you about the enthusiasm he has for what he does. His response to an open-ended question will provide you with a lot more information than using *directed questions* early on in the interview. If you listen carefully, the doctor will tell you how organized he is in his thinking. You will learn how he interacts with you as a person. Listen *between the words*. Get a sense of the person you are dealing with.

Once you have a general idea of how his concierge practice runs, you can start to ask the doctor those directed questions. Concierge practices vary widely. Find out the specifics. Some directed questions that you may want to consider would include:

- How are your routine office visits handled?
- Do you offer same-day appointments?
- What is the nature of your annual physical exam and health assessment?

- How many concierge patients do you have? Is this a small practice, in which the doctor cares for only 100 patients, or does he manage 500 or 600 patients on the plan?
- Who covers your medical practice when you are out-of-town or on vacations?
- Will you take care of me if I need hospitalization?
- Where do you have hospital privileges?
- What is the cost of the program? Is the fee paid in one lump sum, or is it spread out in monthly or quarterly payments?
- How do I reach you in case of an emergency?
- Can you help me in areas of wellness?
- Can you assist me in designing an exercise program?
- Can you help me tailor a nutritional program to meet my needs? Can you help me with weight loss? If not, can you make referrals to help me get this information?
- How do you handle referrals to specialists? (i.e., does he know and choose his specialists carefully, does he talk to them about you before your visit, etc.?)
- Is a stress test part of your initial comprehensive assessment? If not, can you refer me to a cardiologist and help me interpret the results?
- Do you accept insurance as part of the fee?
- Do you accept Medicare assignment as part of the fee?
- Do you make house calls if necessary?
- Can you make any initial recommendations regarding special needs that I may have, such as dealing with chronic heart disease, infertility/pregnancy, or substance abuse?
- Do you offer concierge services for the whole family? Do you care for children?

You don't have to necessarily cover all of these questions. Just ask those that are important to you.

What to Look for in a Doctor

First and foremost, the doctor should be a competent clinician. Most concierge physicians have brochures that highlight their education, training, and areas of special expertise. If this information is not readily available in a brochure, you will want to ask several key questions:

- Which medical school did you go to?
- Where did you do your residency training?

- How long have you been in practice?
- Are you board-certified in your specialty?
- Could I please see a copy of your curriculum vitae?
- How do you keep up-to-date with the challenging task of continuing medical education?

Equally important, you will want to know if this doctor will be a good personality match for you. Is there good chemistry between you and the doctor during the interview? To get a sense of this intangible factor, you will have to rely on your instincts and people skills. Listen to your gut. Do you feel comfortable when talking to the doctor?

We all have different personality styles. A doctor whom one person describes as "direct and honest" may be described by another as "cold and clinical." However, certain characteristics are generally important to all patients:

- Does the doctor listen when you speak during the interview?
- Does he make eye contact?
- Does he allow you to talk and complete your thoughts before responding?
- Does he seem empathetic?
- Does he walk his talk? If the doctor tells you that health and wellness are stressed in his practice, does he look fit and healthy himself?

If you are *only* interested in crisis care medicine, the way that a doctor approaches wellness and optimal human functioning may be less important to you. However, if you believe in the concepts that I have put forth in this book, I would suggest that you find someone who practices what he preaches.

A List of Services

Ask for a written list of services that the doctor provides. Depending on the cost of the program and the number of patients he has, there can be wide differences in the types of services that are offered. Some of the broad services that are offered by concierge doctors include:

- Twenty-four hours per day, seven days per week access to the physician via cell phone or beeper
- Guaranteed same-day appointments
- House calls, where appropriate

- Emergency room and hospital visits
- Wellness care
- Exercise and fitness consultations
- Nutritional consultations
- Blood draws performed in the doctor's office
- Annual executive physicals
- Screening and cancer risk assessments appropriate to the age and sex of the patient
- Prompt telephone feedback following diagnostic tests
- Prompt referral to a strong network of specialists. Some doctors will even accompany a patient to see a specialist when it is appropriate

Patient References

I offer personal references to anyone considering my concierge practice. Some prospective patients find it helpful to talk with a person who has already been on the plan for a few years. If this is important to you, ask the doctor for the names of a couple of patients who may be willing to speak with you.

The Contract

Before you leave the office, ask for a copy of a sample contract. All concierge doctors have contracts with their patients. The contract tells you what you are getting for your money. It tells you what services are offered, how much the plan costs, and how the contract can be terminated by either party.

I always tell my patients, "I am not a contract person. The doctor–patient relationship is founded on trust. If the relationship goes south, there is not a contract in the world that will save it." However, paying a retainer to a physician is a financial investment. It is important to know what you are getting for your retainer fee. This is no different than having a written understanding with an attorney, an accountant, or any other paid professional consultant.

In developing my contract, I made a list of all of the services that I offered. I then gave that list to my attorney and said, "Make this readable for my patients in contract form. I don't want a lot of legalese in the contract. I don't want to start off a relationship with my patient using a cold legal document. Just let my patients know what it is that they are getting for their money and what obligations each party has to the other."

The reason that you receive a contract in concierge medicine is that *you* are actually paying for your own medical care. Unlike third-party payer arrangements, you are spending your own money for your medical care. Your previous doctors signed contracts with the insurance companies and HMOs that paid for your care. Since you are now paying for your medical care, you are in the position to read and request any modifications in the contract. I always tell my patients, "If there is something in the contract that you do not like, tell me about it."

AN IMPORTANT WORD ON WELLNESS SERVICES

No doctor can be all things to all people. Some emphasize wellness more than others. However, health and wellness guidance is fundamental to comprehensive medical care.

As I was writing this book, one of my internal medicine colleagues said to me, "Steve, not all concierge doctors help their patients with exercise and nutritional information. Some doctors still have deficiencies in these areas. Some do not even take care of themselves."

This is a valid point. My response is that *if the demand for wellness services comes from the patient, it will change the way the doctor practices.* If you are seeing the world's greatest cardiologist for a stent placement in your coronary artery, it makes no difference if he emphasizes wellness. He is only doing a procedure on you. All you want from him is the best technical skills that money can buy. On the other hand, a concierge physician is your primary care doctor. He is not only a diagnostician; he is an educator. He will become your healthcare advisor and consultant. Concierge doctors are generalists. They must understand the entire body and how it functions optimally. They must understand health as well as disease.

One of my patients, an overweight cardiologist, called me up one day and said, "I need your help. I've just been diagnosed with type 2 diabetes. I need to lose weight and get in shape. In addition, I told one of my patients last week that he needed to lose weight for his heart. The guy looked at me, pointed at my belly and said, 'And what about you?' I had no credibility!" The cardiologist took my advice. I wrote a program for him. He started exercising. He lost 35 pounds. He got rid of his diabetic medications. He looks and feels better. He now has more credibility with his patients. Success!

It is my hope that this book will help patients, as well as some unhealthy doctors, to understand that there is *no* replacement for exercise and good nutrition in their lives.

It is my strong professional belief that your exercise and nutritional programs should be directed by your personal physician. If your doctor does not presently have the skills to help you do this, he should learn to develop these skills. This is the role of the primary care medical provider. Since time is not a limiting issue in concierge medicine, there is no reason for failing to provide assistance to patients in these areas.

Who am I to tell other concierge doctors that they must address exercise and nutrition with their patients? Isn't this a little arrogant? I am just emphasizing the obvious. All doctors must keep up with important medical advances. It is our duty to our patients. Over the past decade there have been several entirely new classes of oral diabetes medications brought to market. There are new forms of insulin that were not available when I graduated from medical school. It would certainly be unprofessional and unethical for doctors to fail to keep up with these new medicines for diabetes. As new information becomes available, doctors must learn to apply that information to patient care.

During this same period of time, articles in the *New England Journal of Medicine*, *Lancet*, and the *Journal of the American Medical Association* (to name just a few) have unequivocally documented that even moderate exercise can prevent or delay the onset of type 2 diabetes. A sedentary lifestyle has been shown to be a risk factor for heart disease *equal* in magnitude to an elevated cholesterol level. A sedentary lifestyle and being overweight increases your risk of cancer. It is no less professional in the year 2008 for a doctor to fail to teach patients about this *medicine called exercise* than it is to ignore new drug therapies.

Exercise is not just a lifestyle issue. Exercise is the most powerful single medicine known to man. This is why I have included exercise as one of the three critical components of optimal health. I have not just slipped this subject into a book on concierge medicine because the subject interests me.

Likewise, in the area of nutrition and diet there is just too much information out there for patients to process on their own. People need a qualified doctor to help them filter that information. Most doctors received only a couple of hours of formal training in nutrition during medical school. However, a doctor's lifelong learning habits can easily be applied to the mastering of this subject.

WHAT IF THERE ARE NO CONCIERGE DOCTORS NEAR YOU?

If there are no concierge physicians in your town, you may want to talk to your own doctor about starting a concierge practice. This is how my concierge practice began seven years ago. Patients came to me and requested the service. It is happening this way all across the country.

In addition to classic concierge practices that have a contract and a formal structure, there are many doctors across the country that are making informal, direct financial arrangements with their patients. Some doctors are dropping insurance plans altogether and simply charging for their services based upon on how much time they spend with you during an office visit. This may be an option for you if you can't find a concierge doctor right away. Talk to your doctor. Be creative. Drive the system to improve.

Many doctors are fearful about making the transition to concierge medicine. It is scary to leave a system that is well known to them, even if that system is oppressive. It is a big step. However, the number of concierge practices has increased hundredfold over the past five years. If you don't have a concierge doctor on your block today, there will be one tomorrow.

CHAPTER 12

How to Get the Best Return on Your Medical Investment

In this final chapter, I'm going to give you some no-nonsense advice on how to get the most out of your medical investment and your relationship with your doctor. Instead of giving you a polite, sanitized list of suggestions, I am going to be honest with you, even at the risk of being politically incorrect. By doing so, I hope to give you some insight into what doctors appreciate from a patient and what they fear. By understanding your physician–partner, you will be in a better position to get more out of the relationship.

I'm going to cover some topics that many people are not so comfortable discussing. I'm going to ask questions like, What really pisses a doctor off? What puts a doctor on the defensive? So what if your doctor is on the defensive? What do doctors say behind closed doors about the "difficult patient"? How can you get your doctor to go the extra mile for you? How do you bring up a sensitive topic with your doctor, something you'd rather die than talk about, like a sexually transmitted disease?

BE AN ACTIVE AND POSITIVE PARTICIPANT IN YOUR CARE

Before we get started with the practical advice, it is worth discussing your approach. Though it may initially sound trite, you will need to become an active participant in the care of your body. This is the only way to get the best return on your medical investment. Many of us were brought up with the notion of the doctor as the ultimate authority figure, someone not to be questioned. Many people feel they should just keep their mouths shut and stay out of the doctor's way. If you have these kinds of feelings, please discard them. Fortunately, the days of the doctor as the stern, authoritarian father figure are over. You need to be an active partner in your own care.

In this new relationship, you will be sharing the responsibility for your healthcare with a trusted medical partner. In practical terms, this means there will be some things only you can do to improve your health. Likewise, there will be things only your doctor can do to help you; things you cannot do on your own. You need to work together as a team.

THE HEALTH PARTNERSHIP AND DIVISION OF LABOR

People working together toward a common goal can create a synergistic relationship that raises their collective IQ, especially if they bring complementary strengths to the table. However, working effectively in any partnership requires the assignment of specific roles and responsibilities to each partner. Partnerships don't work very well by simply drawing up lists and dividing up the chores equally. I am going to offer suggestions for better defining your role as patient-partner as well as your doctor's role.

In general, your doctor will serve as diagnostician. Once a diagnosis has been made, he will also present the most effective treatment options for your consideration. Treatment options may include drugs, surgery, referral to specialists, and other modalities such as physical therapy. In addition, your doctor should be a clearinghouse for medical information, and a motivator and health educator. It is his job to stay on top of the most recent medical information and to apply that information in the areas of diagnosis, treatment, and the prevention of disease.

Your job is to report any problems or concerns that you have about your health to your doctor. You should avoid being passive and instead ask lots of questions, even if this feels awkward in the beginning. You should read up and take an active role in understanding any medical problems you develop. You should take advantage of your doctor's working knowledge of medicine and get answers to the questions generated from your reading. You should keep copies of important parts of your own medical records. And of course you should be proactive in optimizing your health by remaining physically active and eating as well as you can.

STARTING WITH THE RIGHT ATTITUDE: PEOPLE ARE LIKE CHRISTMAS TREES . . .

As one of my favorite patients once said, "People are like Christmas trees, there's always one side better left facing the corner." We all have missing branches. We all can be ugly under some circumstances. However, if you give yourself permission to be ugly around your doctor on a regular basis, you may get pigeonholed as a "difficult patient." This will not help you get the most out of your doctor, and it could even be detrimental to your care.

The first thing you can do to foster a strong partnership with your doctor is to start with the right attitude. Be positive, as you would at the beginning of any important relationship. Try to be at your best during visits. Approach this endeavor as the *working partnership* that it is.

What's the wrong attitude? Do not take "concierge" literally just because you are paying the doctor directly for his services. As an example, I once had a patient ask me if I was going to be at the hospital at 8:00 A.M. when he would arrive before back surgery just to check him in. "No," I said. "There's no need. Your surgeon will talk with you before the operation. I'll spend that time getting other things done [seeing other patients, honing my skills] and come see you right after the surgery to make sure all went well." He insisted on two visits. He ultimately left my practice.

Though you should not have to change your personality for *anyone*, especially your doctor, this does not mean that it is a good idea to display all of your negative attributes to your physician. I've had patients tell me that their previous doctor "loved them" even though they were "a pain in the ass." I conferred with such patients' previous doctors and learned that this was never the case. Though some people see their doctor as a parental figure with whom they are free to act out, doctors are not like parents. They will not love you no matter how you behave. Your doctor is much more like a partner, with whom mutual respect and consideration are important ingredients for a good working relationship.

For reasons I'll explain in a moment, it is in your best interests to be reasonable and appreciative of your doctor's efforts as often as you can. This just makes sense with any relationship. A sincere thank you when your doctor goes above and beyond the call of duty to help you will mean far more to him than any amount of money you pay. Most doctors really care about their patients and have a need to feel that they've made a difference. Build a positive history with your doctor. If you then lose your temper or composure on some occasion when you are at your worst, the relationship's solid foundation will hold steady.

The Difficult Patient and the Fear of Litigation

Please understand that what I am about to tell you was not written to vent the frustrations doctors have taking care of difficult people. The purpose is to make you aware of what may compromise a potentially good doctor-patient relationship and prevent you from getting the greatest return on your medical investment.

When patients act up or are unreasonable, when they expect perfection for perfection's sake, when they show anger and act self-important, they are labeled by the doctor or his staff as "difficult." Though she may not say so, your doctor will likely be put on the defensive by such behavior. In many cases, people who act inappropriately have major personality disorders, substance abuse issues, or other psychiatric problems. Doctors are trained to read people and diagnose psychiatric troubles. However, due to the litigious environment in which doctors must now practice, any aggressive behavior directed at a physician immediately raises a red flag. The doctor asks herself, "Is this the kind of patient that I can trust, or is this the kind of person who would sue me at the drop of a hat?"

Let me give you the inside scoop: what doctors dislike most in their careers is a lawsuit, even if frivolous, for bogus suits still have to be defended. Surveys of physicians show that a medical malpractice suit is considered one of the most painful experiences of their professional lives.

Even if the doctor does not comment on your bad behavior, it registers in his mind. He becomes defensive. If your doctor feels put on the defensive, it can compromise your care because *it is impossible for anyone to think creatively while they are fending off a perceived threat*. If your doctor is worried that you are a litigious person, his thoughts are to some degree redirected. He is distracted from the focus of addressing your optimal health, for he is now concerned about his own backside.

A defensive doctor is likely to have one of two reactions. He may think of a way to get you out of his practice. Or he may carry a heightened sense of potential litigation throughout the relationship and inadvertently try to protect himself by reducing the smallest chance of error, which could mean ordering excessive tests such as CT scans or blood tests even though the probability of a serious problem is quite low. He may send you to see specialists you don't necessarily need. He may overthink your every complaint, which is not a good idea. These kinds of defensive behaviors result in bad medicine for you.

WHEN SOMETHING GOES WRONG WITH YOUR BODY: HOW TO REPORT A MEDICAL COMPLAINT TO YOUR DOCTOR

Let's talk about how you can communicate more effectively with your physician. People visit the doctor for several reasons. You may be due for your annual physical exam or need a routine follow-up for management of your high blood pressure. However, the most common reason to visit the doctor is a specific complaint or set of new symptoms. This is what a physician refers to as the patient's "chief complaint" during any medical encounter.

Given our easy access to medical information on the Internet, it is very common for patients to start reading on their own as soon as they develop a new symptom. Especially in a time when getting a doctor's appointment can be difficult, patients often start with a little medical sleuthing of their own. However, reading about symptoms may not be the most effective use of your time and can even be counterproductive. Let me illustrate with a little story.

Several years ago, I received a call from the wife of a patient. She said, "Dr. Knope, I'm very worried about my husband. He's been experiencing several hours of severe abdominal pain. I told him to get into the hot shower while I tried to figure out what was wrong with him on the Internet. He's in there writhing in pain and I think he's probably having a gallbladder attack. He can barely stand up. What do you think I should do?" Hmmm. . . . I suggested that she bring her husband to the ER immediately. Twenty minutes later, in the ER, after relieving his pain, we determined that he was experiencing one of the most painful conditions known to man: the passage of a kidney stone. Happily, the couple is still married.

The moral of the story is to avoid being your own diagnostician by trying to find a disease that corresponds with your symptoms. Let your doctor do this. This should be what he does best. Let him be the diagnostician. It is your job to contact him immediately for any serious complaints and to report those symptoms as accurately as possible. One of the problems of reading about a disease and concluding that you've reached the right diagnosis is that it tends to cloud what you tell your doctor. It may actually take the doctor longer to correct your erroneous diagnosis than if you'd just reported the unadulterated symptoms in the beginning.

Most symptoms, such as chest pain or frequent urination, have several possible causes. This is what a doctor calls the "differential diagnosis" for a given complaint. Chest pain, for example, can be due to coronary artery disease, a blood clot to the lung, spasm of the esophagus, dissection of the aorta, or more benign causes, such as muscle strain or acid reflux. Your cluster of symptoms helps the doctor narrow this differential diagnosis to a few possibilities.

When you see a doctor for a new problem, you should report your symptoms in your own words. Just tell your doctor what you are experiencing. If you feel like your "chest is in a vice," simply say that. If you feel a "knifelike pain" in your abdomen, use those words. Doctors have been trained to translate your words into medical diagnoses. About 90 percent of the time, the diagnosis comes from what the patient tells the doctor, long before any fancy test results are back.

I'd Rather Die Than Tell the Doctor about . . .

Earlier in the book, I described the "doorknob syndrome." Not infrequently, patients schedule a visit for a very personal problem and then can't bring themselves to tell the doctor until they are ready to exit the room. Sometimes they are so embarrassed that they don't even mention their problem at all!

Despite the fact that patients intellectually know that doctors are trained not to be judgmental, this does not always register on an emotional level, especially when the problem is one's own. It is easy to recognize the anguish and needless guilt in a patient's eyes when he's about to tell me something he believes involves some moral failing or sign of personal weakness. I've even had more than one doctor bow his head in shame as he comes to me for help with a very personal problem.

Here's my advice on how to handle these difficult situations. Just say something like, "You know, Dr. Smith, I find this very difficult to talk about, but I think I may have contracted a sexually transmitted disease." There, it's out—done! What a relief! Let your doctor take it from there. Just acknowledge that it is difficult for you to talk about your problem, and then let it out. Like a shot, it is over in a matter of seconds. This approach works much better than the old chestnut, "Doctor, I have this friend who has a sore on his penis. What should he do?" Once the doctor hears the opening words that you have a sensitive issue to discuss, this is his cue to address your problem in a nonjudgmental and supportive manner.

It may be helpful to remind yourself that doctors are trained scientists. They know perfectly well that we all have body parts like genitalia or anuses that can suffer from disease and that our bodies can sometimes exude odd noises, smells, or fluids. We no longer live in the dark ages, where illness was treated by punishing the village witch. Part of our job description involves not placing moral judgments on viruses, sexual preferences, or other behaviors that society or certain groups might categorize as sinful or immoral. If your doctor allows his own moral or religious beliefs to interfere with your care or tells you to stop by the confessional on the way to the pharmacy, find another doctor.

READ AND BE ACTIVE

Once a firm diagnosis of a new medical problem has been made, this is the time to start educating yourself. From my perspective, it is much easier to care for a patient who understands his disease than one who says, "You're the doctor," and leaves everything up to me. I strongly encourage most of my patients to read about their problems from reputable sources, and I encourage you to do the same. The one exception to this general rule is when I believe reading on the patient's part will only increase their anxiety. For example, if I have a patient who is anxious to begin with and worries about the worst case scenario with every new problem, I will actually suggest that they stop going to the Internet. Once you have generated a few questions from your reading, go back to your doctor and get those questions answered. Increase your breadth and depth of knowledge over time. This approach will help you become a more educated and active partner.

If you are going to read about medicine, you will want to make sure that you do not waste precious time by ingesting garbage. Make sure that what you read has real substance. Before you put any information into your brain, check that it comes from a reliable source. Medical texts, scientific journals, and Web sites of legitimate medical organizations are usually reliable sources. Advertisements, oddball Websites, TV medical shows, and Aunt Tillie who has lived to 103 and is still going strong on snuff and moonshine are not reliable sources.

Although medical information on the Internet is easily accessible, much of this information is unfiltered. By this I mean that it has not necessarily been peer-reviewed by doctors or other healthcare professionals. Unlike a published textbook from a reliable source, medical information on the Internet may not have been edited at all. Bad information is particularly prevalent on Web sites that cater to difficult problems with which the medical profession has had little success, such as the treatment of fibromyalgia, ADHD, or other conditions whose doors are wide open to a lot of speculation. Other red flags include Web sites that use the word "cure" when that term is not generally applied to the disease. Look for a money trail. If the Web site is selling anything or directs you to PayPal for an untested supplement for chronic fatigue, save your money and get your medical information elsewhere. A good strategy for medical reading is to stick with reliable Web sites that are designed to translate complex medical issues into understandable language. Below are three Web sites to which I often refer my patients:

Healthfinder (www.healthfinder.gov)
WebMD (www.webmd.com)
The National Institutes of Health (www.nih.gov)

If you are comfortable with medical terminology or have a scientific background, you may want to do additional research by exploring individual medical articles. A good place to start is Entrez PubMed (www.pubmed.gov). Simply type in your keyword and begin a literature search. Again, after you've done your reading, follow up with your physician during your next visit to discuss your questions.

WHAT YOU'LL HAVE TO DO ON YOUR OWN

If you accept the idea that there are in fact three critical components to healthcare, you have already realized that two of them will require some work on your part. Without your action, you will have only one of the three components and will not get the greatest return on your medical investment. You should exercise regularly, preferably using a program that has been designed for you with the help of your doctor. As often as you can, you should use the dietary strategies you have discussed with your doctor.

Though I've said this before, it is worth reiterating in this final chapter. Action on your part is the key. Many patients in my practice have gone through the process of creating a dietary plan and writing an exercise program with me, only to discard these plans because "they couldn't find the time." If this happens to you, don't despair. Just get back on track and try to reestablish new, healthier patterns that you *can* stick to.

If life has gotten in the way by robbing you of time you would have liked to use for exercise, recommit and start over the next day. Attempts at lifestyle changes often occur in fits and starts, so don't be too hard on yourself when bad habits return.

Multiple studies have shown that lifestyle changes can reduce all causes of mortality, including from cancer, by up to 30 to 40 percent. Your doctor can offer few things that will provide a similar return on investment.

Follow Good Professional Advice

Gee, now that really sounds like a brilliant piece of advice! So why would I even say this? As the dean of my undergraduate college once said, "There is a reason that there are signs in the New York subways that read, 'No spitting.' It is not because people don't spit on the platform." Similarly, I remind you to follow your doctor's advice, because many otherwise intelligent people do just the opposite. Let me share an example.

I follow standard guidelines for colon cancer screening in my practice. Three times in my career, I have had patients develop colon cancer after refusing, on many occasions, to even consider a colonoscopy. In one case, in which my patient was fortunately cured of her disease, she told me the following at the end of her treatment: "If anyone in your practice ever refuses a colonoscopy, please give them my phone number. The test was really no big deal. In retrospect, all of the reasons I declined the test were irrational. If I can save anyone from having to go through what I did, I would love to help. I was foolish, and it nearly cost me my life."

People often ignore good medical advice because they are in denial about the significance of their symptoms or the gravity of their medical problems. Denial can provide short-term psychological protection from anxiety, but the long-term physical and emotional consequences are not worth the self-deception. All too often, I will advise a patient to follow a course of action to prevent a stroke or some other catastrophe, and he will quip, "Hey, doc, we all have to die of something." True enough. However, without having the experience of watching someone drool in a nursing home after a stroke for untreated high blood pressure, you can't possibly anticipate the consequences of such a cavalier approach to your most precious asset.

My advice is as follows: If your doctor gives you some advice that he says is important, listen carefully. Consider his recommendations seriously. If he looks you in the eye and tells you that he strongly recommends a specific course of action, listen even more carefully. If you are not sure about the reliability of his advice, get a second opinion. But don't just shrug off his advice and hope for the best.

Write Down Your Healthcare Objectives and Keep a Log

The creation of optimal health is not unlike the process of pursuing excellence in any form. The best way to go about it is to set goals, develop a plan, and follow through with it. If you put pen to paper and write down your goals, the chance of you reaching your goals will be greater.

I suggest you buy an inexpensive notebook or folder that you dedicate to your healthcare. If you prefer, keep notes on a word processor and scan your medical reports into your computer.

Record the objectives of your initial visit with your new concierge doctor. Consciously decide what it is you are trying to accomplish. Make brief notes about your follow-up visits over time. Note any responses to treatment that you have, as well as any side effects from drugs. Keep track of how you are doing with your exercise and nutritional programs. You will be amazed at how this process of putting things in writing will help keep you focused on your goals.

Your health goals will change over time. As problems are solved and old goals are reached, set new goals and objectives.

Keep a Copy of Your Medical Reports and Labs

Your medical records are legally yours to see, should you desire to do so. Most medical charts are composed of progress notes written by the doctor, laboratory reports, X-ray reports, EKGs, and correspondence from specialists, as well as hospital records. I do not offer my progress notes to my patients unless they ask to see them. Progress notes document the problems addressed during each visit, along with treatment plans, and much of this is written in medical terminology. However, I do offer to give my patients copies of all of their diagnostic studies, and I help them interpret the results. If you have an MRI of your brain, ask for a copy of the report and understand what it shows. If you have a CT scan of your chest, get the report and read it yourself.

After a doctor orders a test, never take the position that "no news is good news." You can't assume that just because you are not called back by the office the test you took was negative. Sometimes labs fail to send reports to the doctor. Sometimes reports are inadvertently filed in the chart without the doctor ever signing off on them. Despite the fact that most doctors have systems to prevent such errors, errors can and still do occur.

Several years ago, a patient transferred his care to me from a busy medical clinic. As I went through his old medical records, I noticed a chest X-ray report from nine months earlier that documented a 4-cm mass in his lung. The patient was never told of this abnormality. The report was filed by a clerk, and the doctor never saw it. I arranged for a biopsy of the tumor and it proved to be a lung cancer. The patient had surgery and is still alive today.

If these kinds of mistakes were rare, I wouldn't even mention them. However, they occur all too commonly. By being active, you can add an additional check and balance to your own healthcare by simply asking to see all of your reports and keeping them on file for future reference.

THE FUTURE OF CONCIERGE AND
PRIVATE MEDICINE

In closing this chapter and book, I would like to congratulate you for taking the first steps in assuming a more active role in your healthcare. Just by reading this book on concierge medicine, you have taken the time to question the quality of your present healthcare and to ask yourself if there might not be a more proactive way to optimize your health and well-being. For this reason, you are not a typical patient or an average person. You probably want more out of life and are willing to consider investing some time, energy, and money to care for your most precious asset.

Medicine in the United States is in a period of great change. Whether or not this movement called concierge medicine will be successful in improving the medical care for a large number of people remains to be seen. What is true is that the model is growing rapidly.

Some experts would argue that the term concierge medicine is already out-of-date. The Society for Innovative Medical Practice Design (SIMPD), of which I am a member, now prefers the term "direct practices," named for the fact that doctors have direct financial arrangements with their patients. However, a rose is still a rose by any other name, and what this movement represents, regardless of what you call it, is a patient contracting directly with his physician for medical care. The goal is to remove the interference caused by the financial conflicts of interest of third-party payers in this important relationship you have with your doctor.

It is not surprising that this phenomenon of concierge medicine would originate in America. We are an independent people. We don't like anyone telling us what to do. This extends to choices in our medical care—we don't want the government or anyone else telling us whom we can see as our doctor or how much time we can spend with him.

As I said in the beginning of this book, concierge medicine is a patient-driven phenomenon. Though some would call concierge doctors mavericks, I would argue that the patients who see concierge physicians are equally strong individualists. Those patients who originally asked me to open my concierge medical practice seven years ago were fiercely independent people and leaders in their own fields of expertise. As problem solvers, they looked at the state of healthcare and posed a simple question: Why not just get rid of the third-party payers and contract directly with the doctor?

What is *not* new about concierge medicine is its focus on the doctor-patient relationship. I suspect this relationship will always be a fundamental human need. The relationship between a doctor and his patient has been the cornerstone of medical care since the age of Hippocrates, ca. 400 B.C. Fast-food medicine, in contrast, has been with us for little more than a couple of decades.

I wish you the best of luck in finding a competent and caring personal physician who can take the time to properly care for you. I hope that this book has in some way enhanced your overall understanding of the current healthcare system and given you some new options for finding a meaningful relationship with a doctor. I hope that the information I've provided on this powerful new medicine called exercise will empower you to lead a longer and more vibrant life. No matter what your chronological age, I hope that you set a goal of lowering your physiological age by optimizing your health and feeling better inside your skin.

With all of the new medical science and technology available in healthcare, all you need is time with a trusted advisor to help you put this information to good use.

Index

About the Author

STEVEN D. KNOPE, M.D., is a board-certified internist and honors graduate of Cornell Medical College. He is a pioneer in concierge medicine, opening one of the first concierge medicine practices in 2000. He has served as Chief of Medicine, Chief of Internal Medicine, and Director of the Intensive Care Unit at Carondelet Medical System in Tucson, Arizona. He is a nationally recognized expert on health, fitness, and nutrition, as well as an accomplished athlete who holds a third-degree black belt in Kenpo Karate and has completed four Ironman triathlons.